BRAIN POWER and NUTRITION

2018 Report

A Special Report published
by the editors of
Tufts Health & Nutrition Letter
in cooperation with
The Friedman School of Nutrition Science and Policy
Tufts University

Brain Power and Nutrition

Consulting Editor: Robin Kanarek, PhD, John Wade Professor, Department of Psychology, Tufts University

Author: David A. Fryxell, Managing Editor, Tufts Health & Nutrition Letter
Group Director, Belvoir Media Group: Jay Roland
Content Director, Belvoir Media Group: Larry Canale
Creative Director, Belvoir Media Group: Judi Crouse
Editor, Belvoir Media Group: Cindy Foley
Production: Mary Francis McGavic

Publisher, Belvoir Media Group: Timothy H. Cole

ISBN 978-1-879620-96-4

To order additional copies of this report or for customer service questions, please call 877-300-0253, or write: Health Special Reports, 535 Connecticut Avenue, Norwalk, CT 06854-1713.

This publication is intended to provide readers with accurate and timely medical news and information. It is not intended to give personal medical advice, which should be obtained directly from a physician. We regret that we cannot respond to individual inquiries about personal health matters.

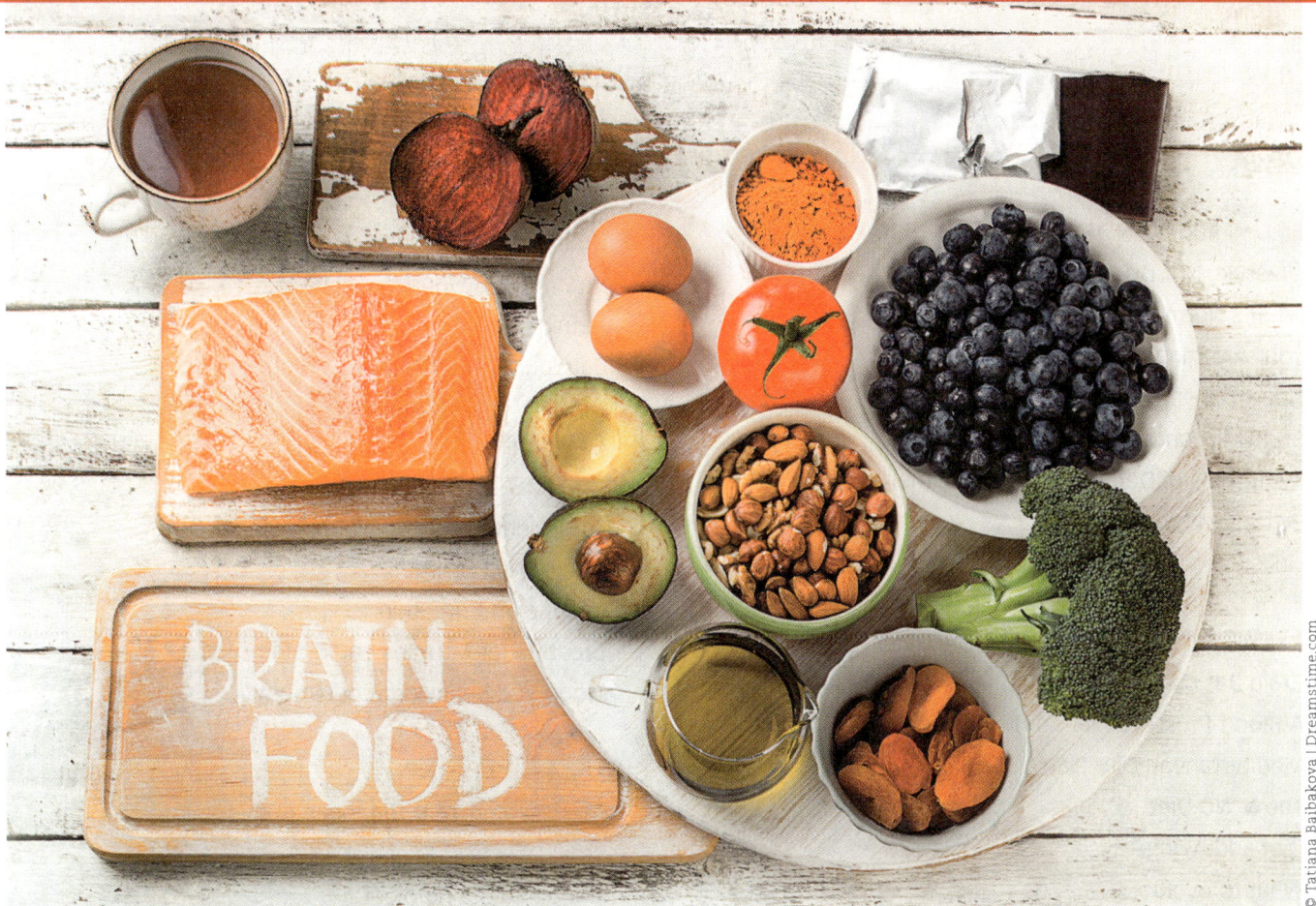

© Tatjana Baibakova | Dreamstime.com

TABLE OF CONTENTS

Never before has so much science been focused on exploring the secrets of the human brain. Grants from the National Institutes of Health to support the Brain Research through Advancing Innovative Neurotechnologies (BRAIN) Initiative now fund research at 125 institutions in the United States and eight other countries. The BRAIN Initiative was launched as a large-scale effort to equip researchers with fundamental insights necessary for treating a wide variety of brain disorders, including Alzheimer's disease. The goal is to catalyze new treatments and cures for devastating brain disorders and diseases that are estimated by the World Health Organization to affect more than 1 billion people worldwide.

Even before the BRAIN Initiative, the National Institute of Neurological Disorders and Stroke estimated that scientists have learned more about the brain in the last decade than in all the previous centuries. The accelerating pace of research in neurological and behavioral science and the development of new research techniques mean we know more than ever before about the brain.

As science learns more about the human brain, the more it becomes clear that the brain is the physical core of who we are. As 17th century French philosopher René Descartes famously expressed it, "I think, therefore I am." That's why when something goes wrong with the brain, as in dementia or simply becoming more forgetful, it's especially frightening.

But the brain is not nearly as mysterious as it was in Descartes's day, and that includes a growing body of research about what individuals can do to protect what makes you you. Science has made dramatic progress not only in understanding the workings of the brain but in preventing and treating disorders that impair its function.

About 50 million Americans suffer from some type of neurological condition related to the brain, from Alzheimer's to Parkinson's disease to approximately 600 other, less well-known brain and neurological disorders. Hope is on the horizon for many of these people, as well as for those who might be threatened by these conditions as they grow older.

As this Special Health Report emphasizes, you don't have to wait to start making dietary and lifestyle changes that contribute to brain health. From overall dietary patterns to specific nutrients, we'll explore the latest thinking on how to protect your own thinking, memory, and mood.

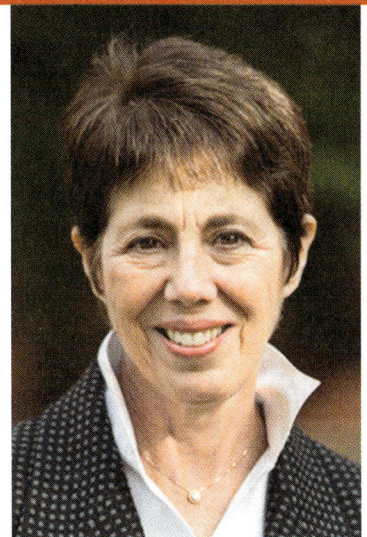

Robin Kanarek, PhD,
John Wade Professor,
Department of Psychology,
Tufts University

Robin Kanarek, PhD,

UNDERSTANDING YOUR BRAIN

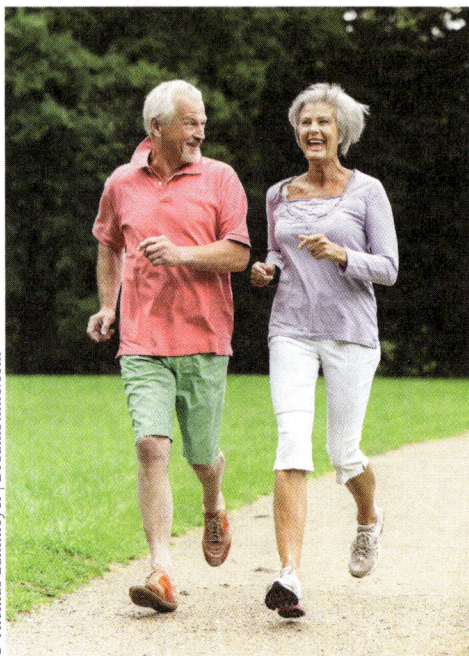

© Thomas Lammeyer | Dreamstime.com

There is surprising good news about the brain and degenerative diseases that can affect it: Predictions that rates of Alzheimer's disease and other dementias will explode as the nation's population ages may have been too pessimistic. According to a study published in 2017 in *JAMA Internal Medicine*, rates of dementia have actually declined in recent years. Moreover, when people do develop dementia, it is striking at an older age.

Research on 21,000 Americans, ages 65 and older, representing all races, education, and income levels, looked at participants in the Health and Retirement Study. The study found that the rate of dementia fell by 24 percent over 12 years, from 11.6 percent in 2000 to 8.8 percent in 2012. Additionally, the average age of dementia diagnosis increased over the same period from 80.7 years old to 82.4.

"The dementia rate is not immutable," says Richard Hodes, MD, director of the National Institute on Aging, which funded the study. "It can change."

A few smaller, more homogeneous studies had shown similar encouraging signs, but an Alzheimer's Association spokesman said experts had previously been reluctant to draw conclusions based on such limited data. Now, Keith Fargo, PhD, director of scientific programs and outreach, says of the new data, "Here is a nationally representative study. It's wonderful news." The findings suggest that roughly a million and a half people ages 65 and older who do not have dementia now would have had it if the rate in 2000 had continued unchanged.

Lifestyle, Not Drugs

What's behind this good news? Experts aren't certain, but it is not due to any breakthroughs in pharmaceutical interventions against Alzheimer's. In fact, even as dementia rates have been declining, the news about medicines to treat the condition has been almost uniformly negative.

"'The history of the results of clinical trials has been a history of disappointment," Dr. Fargo acknowledges. The FDA has approved only four drugs for the treatment of Alzheimer's disease—donepezil (Aricept), galantamine (Razadyne), memantine (Namenda), and rivastigmine (Exelon) Thus far, clinical trials using these drugs have had a 99 percent failure rate, Since 2003, only one new Alzheimer's therapy, Namzanic—a combination of two previously approved drugs, donepezil and memantine—has won federal approval.

Instead, experts on aging believe that improved understanding of the brain, coupled with a population better informed about health and nutrition, can help reduce the toll of Alzheimer's and dementia as the nation ages. Evidence shows, for example, that people who take steps to control their blood pressure and cholesterol have a lower incidence of dementia.

Other research suggests that it's never too early to start taking better care of your brain. A 2015 study published in the journal *Brain* reported that the changes in the brain associated with Alzheimer's disease may be detectable years before the onset of the disease, even in people as young

BOX 1-1

as 20. The findings imply that Alzheimer's disease is truly a lifelong process and that preventive interventions may need to begin much earlier.

What's Normal?

It's true that occasional lapses in memory occur more frequently as people get older. Memory loss and other signs of cognitive decline are not inevitable, however. The serious cognitive losses associated with Alzheimer's disease and other types of dementia are not natural parts of aging. Forgetting where you put your car keys or slipping on a person's name is normal; putting your keys in the stove or being unable to recognize your grandchildren is not.

While some risk factors for Alzheimer's and other forms of dementia, such as genetics, are beyond your control, the good news is that there is much you can do to preserve and even improve your "brain power."

Your Amazing Brain

The human brain weighs only about three pounds, yet manages to carry on thousands of chemical reactions every second. Although on average the brain makes up only two percent of a person's body weight, your hard-working brain consumes 20 percent of the oxygen you breathe and 20 percent of the energy you take in from food.

To understand how the brain works, think of it like a baseball team (see "The Brain," Box 1-1). Each specialized part of the brain—like the pitcher, catcher, shortstop, and others on a baseball team—performs a specific job. If any one part of the team fails, such as a pitcher serving up a "gopher" ball or a shortstop bobbling a fielding play, a whole inning can be lost.

The hindbrain, which includes the upper spinal cord, brainstem, and cerebellum, controls the body's vital functions, such as heart rate and breathing. The cerebellum also manages movement and the actions your body has "memorized," such as swinging a golf club or playing the piano. The midbrain, the uppermost part of the brainstem, controls some of your reflexes and is part of the process that coordinates eye movements and other voluntary motions.

Where Thinking Happens

The cerebrum, part of the forebrain that is located at the top of the brain, is the site of those activities we broadly call "thinking." When you read a newspaper, play bridge, write an email, or recognize a friendly face, your cerebrum is at work. It stores your memories and enables you to plan and carry out those plans—what cognitive scientists call "executive function."

You've probably also heard the terms "left brain" and "right brain," which refer to the cerebrum's two hemispheres. Each hemisphere specializes in certain kinds of tasks the brain performs: Typically, the right side of the brain is responsible for more creative functions, while the left hemisphere performs grammar, vocabulary, and logical chores. However, both hemispheres actually contribute to many of these processes.

Each hemisphere controls the opposite side of the body, with nerve signals crisscrossing between the brain's right hemisphere and your left

THE BRAIN

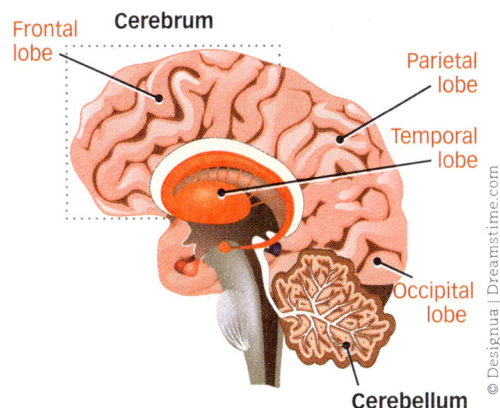

Different parts of the brain are responsible for different aspects of thought, mood, and behavior. For example, the frontal lobes are responsible for speech, emotion, behavior, movement, intellect, and planning, while the temporal lobes handle personality, memory, and language.

hand, and vice versa. So when one side of the brain is damaged, such as by a stroke or traumatic injury, it's the opposite side of the face and body that may droop or be paralyzed.

Lobes at Work

The lobes of the brain handle additional specific tasks. The frontal lobes, located behind the forehead, take charge of planning, weighing alternatives, and envisioning possible consequences. One way they seem to do this is by temporarily storing options and thoughts you are considering ("Hamburgers tonight … or pizza?") in working memory.

At the back of each frontal lobe, a motor area helps manage voluntary movement. Nearby, in the left frontal lobe, Broca's area is responsible for turning your thoughts into words.

The parietal lobes, located behind the frontal lobes, handle sensory input and are also important for math and reading. The occipital lobes, at the back of the brain, process images from the eyes. The temporal lobes, located under the parietal and frontal lobes, perform similar chores with input from the ears, as well as integrating sensory information and memories.

Deeper in the Brain

Farther inside the brain, several interior structures, including the thalamus and basal ganglia, act as mediators between the cerebral hemispheres and the spinal cord. The hypothalamus, also in the interior of the brain, is important for maintaining your sleep/wake cycle, food and water intakes, and responses to stress.

Deep inside the brain, the hippocampus is important to your brain far out of proportion to its size. Acting as a sort of a hard drive for your memories, the hippocampus "indexes" your memories and sends them to other parts of the brain when needed.

Grey and White Matter

You've likely also heard of the brain's "grey matter," which refers not to the whole brain but rather only to the coating of the surface of the cerebrum and cerebellum. This coating is about an eighth of an inch thick—sort of like the bark on a tree. Formally called the cerebral cortex—from the Latin for "bark"—it really is grey. That's because the cortex lacks a white insulating material called myelin that is found elsewhere in the brain; this myelin sheath allows electrical impulses to transmit quickly and efficiently along nerve cells.

Myelin makes most of the brain white, so you will also see references to "white matter." The cortex also is famously wrinkled, and these folds serve a purpose: Much of the brain's information processing occurs in the cerebral cortex, and its wrinkles create more surface area for this processing.

Neurotransmitters

All the various parts of your brain, large and small, communicate with one another and with the nervous system throughout your body using tiny electrical impulses along with chemical signals called neurotransmitters.

BOX 1-2

Zooming in to the microscopic level, thinking and other functions of the brain and nervous system are performed by cells called neurons (see "Message Passing Across a Synapse," Box 1-2). An adult brain contains approximately 100 billion neurons, with branches that connect at more than 100 trillion junction points called synapses.

Neurons consist of several parts: the cell body, which includes the nucleus and most of the molecules that keep the neuron alive; dendrites, which act like telegraph wires bringing data from other neurons; and axons, which carry the signals away to other cells in the body.

When a neuron is activated, a small difference in electrical charge—called an action potential—is created by the concentration of electrically charged atoms (ions) on the cell membrane of an axon. This charge zooms rapidly down the axon until it comes to the end junction point, the synapse. In most neurons, the action potential then causes the release of a neurotransmitter. This chemical message travels across the minute gap of the synapse. On the other side of the synapse, the neurotransmitter binds to receptors on the dendrites of the receiving neuron. The signal then continues in the same way from one neuron to the next, via electrical charges and neurotransmitters.

Ultimately, when the message reaches its destination, a neurotransmitter might set off a fresh chain of messages along the neurons. Or the result could be the stimulation of another kind of cell, such as those found in glands. When your body sends a "fight or flight" signal, for example, neurotransmitters wind up triggering the adrenal gland.

When Neurotransmitters Go Awry

Most of the time in healthy people, the messaging of neurotransmitters proceeds without any glitches and without our even being aware of what's happening. When things go wrong, however, malfunctions of these neurotransmitters are associated with certain diseases of the brain. For example, a characteristic feature of Alzheimer's disease is a reduction in levels of acetylcholine, a neurotransmitter involved in memory.

Parkinson's disease is linked to low levels of dopamine, a neurotransmitter important in controlling movement. When the body lacks adequate amounts of dopamine, the result can be tremors, shaking, stiffness, and other symptoms characteristic of Parkinson's disease.

Dopamine also affects the reward systems in the brain and assists in the flow of information to the front of the brain, where thinking and emotions reside. So research has also suggested that low levels of dopamine or issues with utilizing dopamine in these parts of the brain might be factors in attention-deficit/hyperactivity disorder (ADHD).

Mental illnesses can also be associated with neurotransmitter problems. For example, another neurotransmitter, serotonin, works to help control functions, such as sleep, mood, and appetite. People who suffer from depression often suffer from lower than normal levels of serotonin. That's why the most commonly prescribed medications to treat depression are called selective serotonin-reuptake inhibitors (SSRIs): They work by blocking the automatic "reuptake" of serotonin, in which the sending neuron recycles the

Message Passing Across a Synapse

Neurotransmitters pass across the synapses between nerve cells, enabling these cells to communicate.

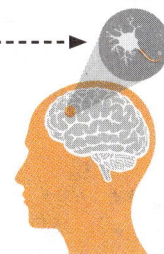

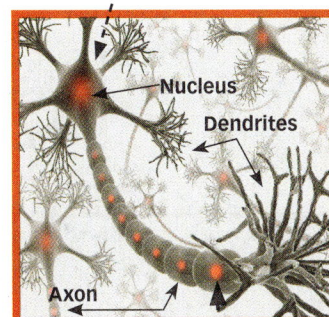

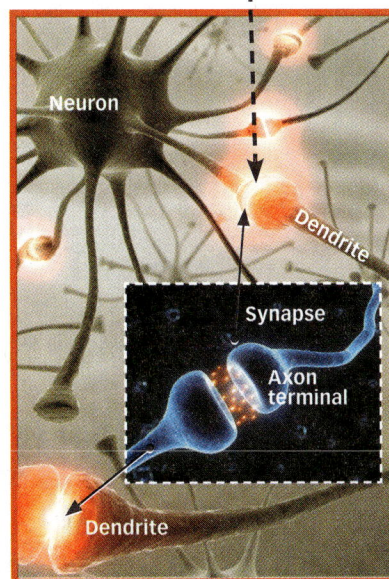

© Ponkrit Uthaikorn | Dreamstime.com

© Kts | Dreamstime.com

© Eraxion | Dreamstime.com

© Kts | Dreamstime.com

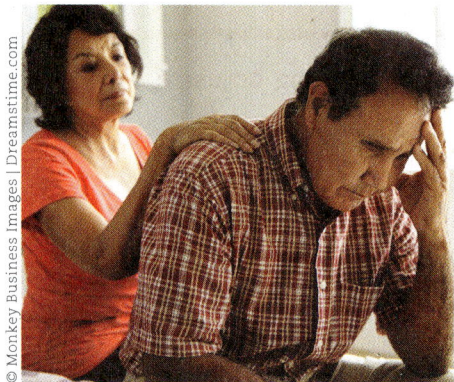

serotonin used to cross a synapse. That leaves more serotonin to bind onto the receiving neuron, encouraging more normal functioning and moods.

Some studies have pointed to a role for inadequate or ineffective amounts of dopamine in the development of another mental illness, schizophrenia.

Neurotransmitters and Alzheimer's

Where other brain conditions may be caused in part by problems with neurotransmitters, Alzheimer's disease also disrupts the normal functioning of these chemical messengers and the cells they affect. The disease damages the brain's communications system by actually destroying synapses and killing neurons.

Some of the FDA-approved medications for the treatment (but not cure) of Alzheimer's disease work by trying to counter these communication breakdowns. According to the Alzheimer's Association, current FDA-approved Alzheimer's drugs support this communication process through two different mechanisms:

▶ Cholinesterase inhibitors (donepezil, galantamine, rivastigmine) work by slowing down the process that breaks down acetylcholine.
▶ Memantine is an NMDA (N-methyl-D-aspartate) receptor antagonist, which works by regulating the activity of glutamate. By partially blocking NMDA receptors, the drug prevents the excess release of glutamate from damaged cells. Too much glutamate lets excess calcium enter cells, which can trigger further damage.

Brain Misconceptions

Contrary to the common misperception that neurons can only form new connections during early brain development, the brain actually continues to change in response to new inputs—a characteristic called plasticity. Even adult brains can form new neuronal connections, strengthen existing ones, or eliminate old ones as you continue to gather new knowledge and experiences. Stimulating neurons can cause them to grow and form new synaptic connections, while those that go without stimulation may weaken.

This plasticity helps explain why practicing a task, such as learning to play a musical instrument, helps a person perform that task better and more efficiently. Doing something over and over again strengthens the synapses involved in that task—like paving a road to make repeated journeys go more smoothly.

Symptoms of Dementia and Alzheimer's

Symptoms of Alzheimer's disease and other forms of dementia occur when things go wrong in the brain. These symptoms of a decline in cognition—what we loosely call thinking and memory—affect a person's ability to conduct everyday activities. The umbrella term for a wide range of such symptoms is "dementia," which is not a specific disease or single condition. The best-known form of dementia, Alzheimer's disease, accounts for 60 to 80 percent of all cases.

The earliest signs of dementia may be what's called mild cognitive impairment (MCI), a stage between normal forgetfulness due to aging and more serious cognitive decline (see "Symptoms of Mild Cognitive Impairment," Box 1-3). Mild cognitive impairment manifests as problems with thinking and memory that do not interfere with everyday activities. People with this condition are often aware that they are showing signs of impairment. Not everyone who develops mild cognitive impairment progresses to Alzheimer's or other dementia.

Symptoms of Dementia

Many of the first symptoms of actual dementia, such as being unable to come up with a word that's on the tip of your tongue or misplacing things, are common in everyday life for people who are perfectly normal. (see "Early Signs of Dementia," Box 1-4). Many of these early signs of actual dementia are also similar to the symptoms of mild cognitive impairment. To be considered dementia, at least two of these core mental functions must be significantly impaired:

- Ability to focus, pay attention
- Communication, language
- Memory
- Reasoning and judgment
- Visual perception

As dementia worsens, symptoms grow more obvious and interfere with the ability to take care of oneself and conduct everyday life. People with severe dementia may no longer be able to perform basic activities of daily living, recognize family members, or even understand language.

Diagnosing Alzheimer's

The earliest stages of Alzheimer's may begin as many as 20 years before the disease is severe enough to be diagnosed. When Alzheimer's strikes relatively younger people, it may not be characterized by the memory problems we associate with the disease. A study published in the November 2015 issue of *Alzheimer's & Dementia* stated that tests for non-memory cognitive problems should not be overlooked when screening for Alzheimer's.

In mild and moderate stages of Alzheimer's, the growing plaques and tangles impair mental functions enough to affect everyday activities and to be noticed by loved ones. This is when the disease is most often diagnosed (see "10 Warning Signs of Alzheimer's," Box 1-5).

Alzheimer's Brain Changes

Unlike dementia in general, Alzheimer's disease is associated with specific changes in the physical condition of the brain. A brain affected by Alzheimer's has far fewer nerve cells and synapses than a healthy brain. The "grey matter" actually begins to shrivel, impairing the ability to process information. The hippocampus, so important to the formation of new memories, shrinks. Fluid-filled spaces within the brain, called ventricles, grow larger.

When reading about Alzheimer's disease, you'll see references to two types of characteristic brain formations, called plaque and tangles. Plaque is formed when pieces of a "sticky" protein called beta-amyloid, which

BOX 1-3

Symptoms of Mild Cognitive Impairment

- Difficulty performing more than one task at a time
- Inability to solve problems or make decisions
- Forgetting recent events or conversations
- Taking longer to perform difficult mental activities

BOX 1-4

Early Signs of Dementia

According to the National Library of Medicine, early symptoms of dementia can include:

- Difficulty performing tasks that take thought, but that used to come easily, such as balancing a checkbook, playing bridge, or learning new information or routines
- Getting lost on familiar routes
- Language problems, such as trouble remembering the name of familiar objects
- Losing interest in things you previously enjoyed; flat mood
- Misplacing items
- Personality changes and loss of social skills, which can lead to inappropriate behaviors

BOX 1-5

10 Warning Signs of Alzheimer's

The Alzheimer's Association lists these early warning signs of Alzheimer's disease.

1. Memory loss that disrupts daily life.
2. Challenges in planning or solving problems.
3. Difficulty completing familiar tasks at home, at work, or at leisure.
4. Confusion with time or place.
5. Trouble understanding visual images and spatial relationships.
6. New problems with words in speaking or writing.
7. Misplacing things and losing the ability to retrace steps.
8. Decreased or poor judgment.
9. Withdrawal from work or social activities.
10. Changes in mood and personality.

For details, see www.alz.org/10signs.

comes from fatty membranes that surround nerve cells, clump together. Scientists suspect that larger plaques may not be as damaging to brain function as smaller clumps of beta-amyloid that block the messaging between the brain's synapses.

Tangles are like traffic jams in your brain. In a healthy brain, parallel strands of "tau" proteins function like highways, carrying essential nutrients. In Alzheimer's patients, tangles of collapsed tau block the orderly flow along the highways that serve the brain. Eventually, the cells deprived of nutrients die.

As these plaques and tangles spread through the grey matter of the brain, Alzheimer's disease progresses. Typically, plaques and tangles strike first in areas important to learning, memory, thinking, and planning.

Picturing the Brain

At one time, the diagnosis of Alzheimer's disease could be definitively confirmed only after death, via autopsy. But today, new imaging techniques make it possible to see the damage the disease causes in a living brain and to better understand how healthy brains function.

More detailed pictures of the brain, without the use of X-rays, can be obtained by magnetic resonance imaging (MRI). This technology takes advantage of the fact that hydrogen atoms in the brain can be affected by rotating a powerful magnet around a person's head; the resulting changes in these atoms' energy levels can be captured to create detailed images. Both CT (computed tomography) and MRI scans are static—like snapshots of the brain.

Links Between Heart and Brain

The brain is fed by one of the richest networks of blood vessels in the body, so changes in your cardiovascular system affect brain function—with important consequences for protecting your aging brain. Every heartbeat carries roughly one-fifth to one-quarter of your blood supply to the brain, and an even greater percentage when your brain is working hard.

Recent research has suggested that a healthy heart and blood pressure in midlife might be associated with brain volume decades later. An observational study of 1,094 participants in the Framingham Offspring cohort compared results from a treadmill test when the volunteers were about age 40 with brain volume almost 20 years later, measured by MRI scans. Participants with initial lower cardiovascular fitness and elevated blood pressure and heart rate responses subsequently averaged smaller brain volumes. Researchers said the findings linked "fitness over the life course to brain health in later life," adding, "Promotion of midlife cardiovascular fitness may be an important step toward ensuring healthy brain aging in the population, especially in pre-hypertensive or hypertensive individuals." Of course, since this was an observational study, it could also be that the association goes the other way, and a healthy brain contributes to cardiovascular health.

> Every heartbeat carries roughly one-fifth to one-quarter of your blood supply to the brain, and an even greater percentage when your brain is working hard.

Blood Vessels and the Brain

Vascular dementia, the second-most common form of dementia after Alzheimer's disease, begins with blood vessel damage in the brain: A stroke or a series of tiny strokes cuts off or restricts the flow of blood to brain cells, interfering with their ability to communicate with other brain cells. That in turn affects everything from your ability to think to your emotions. Vascular dementia may manifest in different ways, depending on which areas of the brain suffer damage.

Blood-vessel changes can also increase the degree of impairment or the speed of cognitive decline in other forms of dementia, such as Alzheimer's, or a condition known as Lewy-body dementia.

Heart-Brain Health

These connections mean that many of the ways in which you can protect your brain also benefit your heart, and vice versa, because a healthy brain depends on a healthy cardiovascular system. Although you can't control some risk factors for Alzheimer's and other dementias, others you can. In particular, you can help protect your brain by improving your cardiovascular health with these steps:

- Keep your blood-cholesterol levels healthy by cutting down on saturated and trans fats and, if prescribed by your doctor, taking cholesterol-lowering drugs, such as statins.
- Replace unhealthy fats with unsaturated fats; current evidence suggests that polyunsaturated fats, found in liquid vegetable oils and nuts, are the most heart-healthy choice, though other benefits have been associated with monounsaturated fats, found in olive and canola oils and avocados.
- Control your blood pressure by reducing salt intake, following a healthy diet (the DASH eating plan is specially formulated to combat hypertension), and taking blood-pressure medications if prescribed by your doctor.
- If you smoke, here's another reason to quit; if you don't smoke, don't start.
- Follow a heart-healthy diet, such as DASH (see above) or a Mediterranean-style diet, which we'll explore in the next chapter.
- Maintain a healthy weight.
- Maintain healthy blood-glucose levels by watching your weight and reducing intake of refined carbohydrates, starches, and sugar to avoid diabetes, which in turn contributes to heart disease.
- Follow exercise guidelines, which generally advise getting 30 minutes a day of at least moderate physical activity on most days of the week. Exercise seems to directly benefit brain health by increasing blood and oxygen flow to brain cells, and benefits your overall cardiovascular system.

As we'll see in the rest of this Special Health Report, smart choices about nutrition and lifestyle can make a big difference. While some things about your aging brain are beyond your control, these simple steps can improve your odds.

PATTERNS FOR BRAIN HEALTH

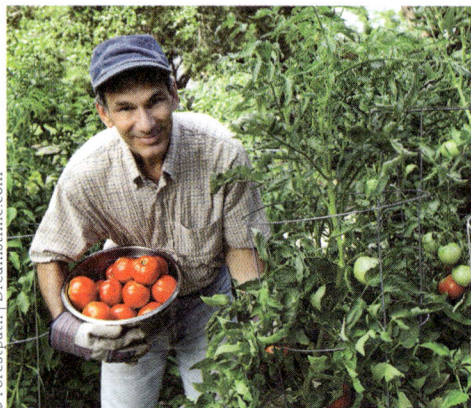

A lthough certain individual foods have frequently been associated with brain health, as we'll see in the next chapter, protecting your brain isn't as simple as eating a few extra blueberries or sipping an occasional cup of green tea. The health of your brain—like your overall health—instead requires a healthy dietary pattern.

Brain Basics

The updated Dietary Guidelines for Americans (DGAs) didn't recommend a single, one-size-fits-all dietary pattern, although several patterns were cited as healthy examples and are included in this chapter. The DGAs did, however, offer a list of what to look for in a healthy dietary pattern—good advice for lifelong healthy eating, as well as a smart start for eating right for your brain. These principles include consuming:

- A variety of vegetables from all of the subgroups—dark green, red and orange, legumes (beans and peas)
- Fruits, especially whole fruits
- Grains, at least half of which are whole grains
- Fat-free or low-fat dairy, including milk, yogurt, cheese, and/or fortified soy beverages
- A variety of protein foods, including seafood, lean meats and poultry, eggs, legumes (beans and peas), and nuts, seeds, and soy products
- Unsaturated oils
- A healthy eating pattern limits saturated fats and trans fats, added sugars, and sodium

A Blood-Pressure Plan for Brain Health

Among the dietary patterns recommended by the DGAs is one that's proven to improve blood pressure, the Dietary Approaches to Stop Hypertension (DASH) eating plan, designed by the National Heart, Lung, and Blood Institute. Following a DASH-style pattern seems to also be good for your brain—not surprising, since cardiovascular health is linked to protecting your brain against strokes and dementia. The DASH regimen is high in fruits, vegetables, and grains, while cutting back on meat, saturated fat, sweets, and salt.

The DASH plan was based on clinical studies that tested the effects of sodium and other nutrients on blood pressure. The first DASH study compared three eating plans: a typical American diet, the typical American diet with added fruits and vegetables, and the DASH plan. People who followed the high fruits and vegetables plan had reduced blood pressure, and those who followed the DASH eating plan experienced even greater drops in blood pressure. A second DASH study examined the effects of restricting sodium, comparing diets with sodium levels of 3,300 milligrams (mg), 2,300 mg, and 1,500 mg per day. (The latest dietary guidelines call for a maximum of 2,300 mg daily.) The greatest blood pressure reduction occurred with the DASH plan that was lowest in sodium. Moreover, the DASH eating plan lowered blood pressure more than the typical Western diet at any of the sodium levels.

Subsequent research has shown that even partly adhering to a DASH plan also pays off for cognitive protection. People whose diets most closely adhered to the DASH pattern scored higher on the Modified Mini-Mental State Examination (MMMSE), a standard cognitive measurement. Re-tested 11 years later, those in the top DASH group scored even higher compared to those in the group least-adherent to the DASH diet.

The results suggest that including whole grains, vegetables, low-fat dairy foods, and nuts in the diet may offer benefits for cognition in later life, researchers commented. They concluded, "We believe that what we have observed is that the total DASH-like diet is greater than the sum of its parts."

Mediterranean Diet Plan

Another heart-healthy dietary pattern that seems to have brain benefits is the "Mediterranean diet" (see "Mediterranean Diet Pyramid," Box 2-1 and "Defining the Mediterranean Diet," Box 2-2). Following this traditional dietary pattern typically consumed in Mediterranean countries has been shown to have cardiovascular benefits. But research shows that the Mediterranean diet also seems to be good for your brain.

Most recently, a study published in the journal *Neurology* reported an association between adherence to a Mediterranean-style diet and brain volume (see "Mediterranean Diet Linked to Bigger Brains," Box 2-3).

An earlier study published in *Neurology* reported that sticking to a Mediterranean-style diet, with more fish and less meat, might help

BOX 2-2

Defining the Mediterranean Diet

Despite the popularity of the term, there's no such thing as an official "Mediterranean diet." When researching the possible benefits of a dietary pattern similar to that traditionally found in areas around the Mediterranean compared to the typical American diet, scientists generally look for:

MORE
- Fruits
- Vegetables
- Legumes
- Grains (mostly whole)
- Fish
- Monounsaturated fats (such as olive oil)
- Nuts and seeds

LESS
- Red meat
- Dairy products
- Saturated fats
- Sweets

ALSO …
- Moderate alcohol consumption, especially of red wine with meals

BOX 2-1

Mediterranean Diet Pyramid

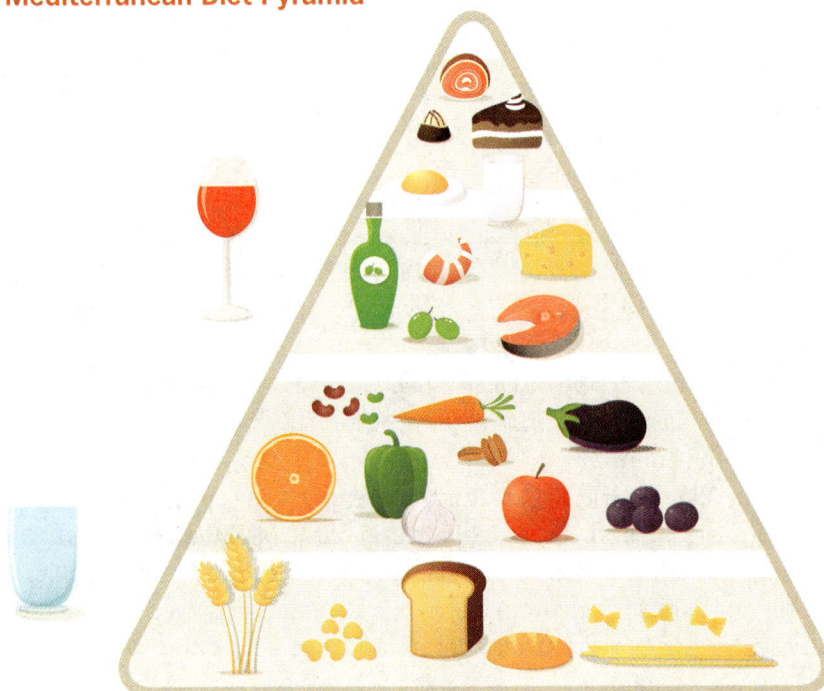

© Yan Batshev | Dreamstime.com

NEW FINDING BOX 2-3

Mediterranean Diet Linked to Bigger Brains

Researchers in Scotland compared the reduction in brain volume over three years among people in their mid-70s who ate more of a Mediterranean diet versus those consuming traditional Scottish fare. The study used a group of Edinburgh residents, born in 1936, who have been followed ever since; scientists asked them to fill out a food diary and have MRI scans of their brains. Among about 400 participants who had scans three years apart, lower adherence to a Mediterranean diet was associated with greater reduction in total brain volume. But those who ate the most fruits, vegetables, olive oil, and other Mediterranean fare, and the least fried food, red meat, and cheese, had about half the expected rate of brain shrinkage. Light-to-moderate drinking—no more than three drinks a day on average for men and two for women—was also part of the healthy pattern.

Neurology, Jan. 4, 2017

keep your brain younger. When cognitively healthy older adults most closely followed a Mediterranean diet, their brains' aging processes slowed by the equivalent of up to five years. The Columbia University study used MRIs to measure the brains of 674 older adults, average age 80, and compared that data to adherence to a Mediterranean eating pattern as gauged by food questionnaires. Those with scores in the half most closely sticking to the pattern had larger brain volumes. The study assigned points to high intake of vegetables, legumes, fruits, cereals, fish, and monounsaturated fatty acids, such as olive oil; a low intake of saturated fatty acids, dairy products, meat, and poultry; and moderate alcohol consumption. When analyzed separately, higher fish intake, lower meat consumption, and moderate alcohol use were also associated with greater brain volumes.

Adding to the Evidence

Individual studies specifically focused on the Mediterranean diet have also added to this evidence. Data on 17,478 participants in the Reasons for Geographic and Racial Differences in Stroke (REGARDS) study, average age 64, revealed that healthy people eating more Mediterranean-style diets were 19 percent less likely to develop cognitive impairment over four years. That meant consuming more fish and plant products while eating less red meat and dairy.

An earlier Columbia University study found that subjects who adhered to a Mediterranean-style eating plan were at lower risk of Alzheimer's disease. The regimen consisted mostly of vegetables, legumes, fruits, whole-grain cereals, and some fish, and was high in monounsaturated fats and low in saturated fat, meat, and dairy. Even after adjusting for demographics and known risk factors, one-third of the individuals in the study who followed the Mediterranean-style diet most closely had about a 40 percent reduced risk of developing Alzheimer's compared to the group with the lowest adherence. Each additional unit of adherence to a Mediterranean diet (measured on a 0-9 scale) was associated with a nine-to-10 percent reduction in Alzheimer's risk.

The MIND Diet

While both the DASH eating plan and a Mediterranean-style diet are associated with brain benefits, a hybrid dietary pattern—called the MIND diet—that combines the best of both with the latest cognitive research may protect memory and thinking even better. A study published in the journal *Alzheimer's & Dementia* in September 2015 offered intriguing evidence of a dietary pattern that seems especially well suited to protecting the brain.

Martha Clare Morris, ScD, of Rush University, and colleagues developed the MIND diet score as a hybrid of the Mediterranean and DASH diets. But it also particularly focuses on "the dietary components and servings linked to neuroprotection and dementia prevention." Many of these components are foods and nutrients we'll look at in depth in the next few chapters.

BOX 2-4

Similar to the Mediterranean and DASH regimens, MIND "emphasizes natural plant-based foods and limited intakes of animal and high saturated-fat foods, but uniquely specifies the consumption of berries and green leafy vegetables."

Differences and Don'ts

There are some differences, too. The MIND diet doesn't specify high fruit consumption other than berries. "Blueberries are one of the more potent foods in terms of protecting the brain," researchers noted, and strawberries have also performed well in past studies of the effect of food on cognitive function.

MIND drops the DASH recommendation for high dairy consumption and calls for only weekly fish consumption, which is lower than recommended in the Mediterranean diet.

The MIND regimen also specifies some dietary don'ts, identifying five unhealthy groups to limit:

- Red meats
- Butter and stick margarine
- Cheese
- Pastries and sweets
- Fried or fast food

The MIND diet includes at least three servings of whole grains, a salad, and one other vegetable every day—along with a glass of wine. It also involves snacking most days on nuts and eating beans every other day or so, poultry and berries at least twice a week, and fish at least once a week. Dieters must limit eating the designated unhealthy foods, especially butter (less than 1 tablespoon a day), cheese, and fried or fast food (less than a serving a week for any of the three), to have a real shot at avoiding the devastating effects of Alzheimer's, according to the study (see "What's Your MIND Score?" Box 2-4).

Diets vs. Alzheimer's

The prospective study used a 144-item food questionnaire to score 923 participants ages 58 to 98, in the Rush Memory and Aging Project, for adherence to each type of diet: MIND, DASH, or Mediterranean-style. Responses were assigned points to score how closely their diets matched each of the three dietary patterns being tested. Participants were initially free of Alzheimer's disease. They were then followed for an average 4.5 years to track who developed Alzheimer's disease; during the study, 144 incident cases of Alzheimer's were diagnosed.

In the study, the MIND diet was associated with a slower rate of cognitive decline—equivalent to 7.5 years of younger age. Those with the highest MIND diet scores were 53 percent less likely to develop Alzheimer's disease than those with the lowest scores.

The lower risk for those most closely following the MIND diet was similar to those with the highest adherence to a Mediterranean diet (54 percent) and the DASH plan (39 percent). But only the top one-third of Mediterranean and DASH scores were associated with lower Alzheimer's risk.

What's Your MIND Score?

The MIND diet score assigns a maximum of one point for each of these components, up to a total of 15 points:

- Whole grains, at least 3 servings/day
- Green leafy vegetables, at least 6 servings/week
- Other vegetables, at least 1 serving/day
- Berries, at least 2 servings/week
- Red meats, fewer than 4 servings/week
- Fish, at least 1 serving/week
- Poultry, at least 2 servings/week
- Beans, at least 3 servings/week
- Nuts, at least 5 servings/week
- Fast/fried food, less than 1 serving/week
- Olive oil as primary oil
- Butter/margarine, less than 1 Tbsp/day
- Cheese, less than 1 serving/week
- Pastries/sweets, less than 5 servings/week
- Alcohol, 1 serving/day

The second-highest third of MIND scores were also associated with lower risk (35 percent), however, suggesting that even modest dietary improvements following the MIND pattern could be beneficial.

Although the observational study was not designed to prove cause and effect, Morris and colleagues noted that the results "suggest that even modest adjustments to the diet may help to reduce one's risk of Alzheimer's disease. For example, the MIND diet score specifies just two vegetable servings per day, two berry servings per week, and one fish meal per week." Those recommendations are much lower and easier to achieve than comparable guidelines in the Mediterranean or DASH plans.

Although more research needs to be done, it makes sense that such a dietary pattern might help make a difference for brain health. "Inflammation and oxidative stress play a large role in the development and progression of Alzheimer's disease," says Tammy Scott, PhD, a scientist at Tufts' HNRCA Neuroscience and Aging Laboratory. "The MIND diet particularly emphasizes foods, such as green leafy vegetables, berries, and olive oil, which are rich in antioxidants and anti-inflammatory agents that may help to protect against dementia and cognitive decline."

BOX 2-5

MyPlate for Older Adults

Fruits & Vegetables

Whole fruits and vegetables are rich in important nutrients and fiber. Choose fruits and vegetables with deeply colored flesh. Choose canned varieties that are packed in their own juices or low-sodium.

Healthy Oils

Liquid vegetable oils and soft margarines provide important fatty acids and some fat-soluble vitamins.

Herbs & Spices

Use a variety of herbs and spices to enhance flavor of foods and reduce the need to add salt.

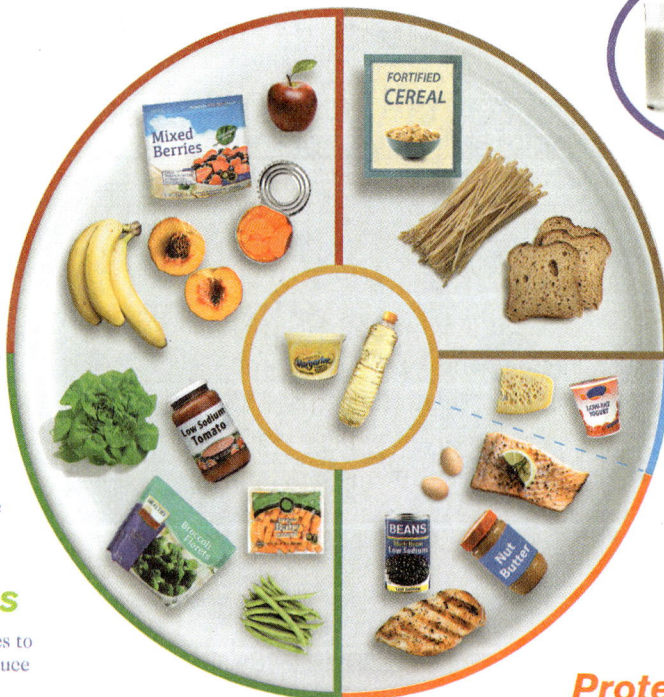

Fluids

Drink plenty of fluids. Fluids can come from water, tea, coffee, soups, and fruits and vegetables.

Grains

Whole grain and fortified foods are good sources of fiber and B vitamins.

Dairy

Fat-free and low-fat milk, cheeses and yogurts provide protein, calcium and other important nutrients.

Protein

Protein rich foods provide many important nutrients. Choose a variety including nuts, beans, fish, lean meat and poultry.

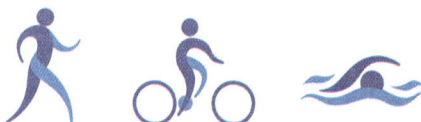

Remember to Stay Active!

Tufts UNIVERSITY   JEAN MAYER USDA HUMAN NUTRITION RESEARCH CENTER ON AGING   HNRCA   AARP Foundation

Diet and Aging

Whether specifically for brain health or overall health, the dietary needs of older adults are differen than those of younger individuals. In March 2016, nutrition scientists at Tufts' Jean Mayer USDA Human Nutrition Research Center on Aging introduced an updated MyPlate for Older Adults (see "MyPlate for Older Adults," Box 2-5), revised to reflect the latest Dietary Guidelines for Americans. This system calls attention to the unique nutritional and physical activity needs associated with advancing years, emphasizing positive choices. It shows how older adults might follow a healthy dietary pattern that builds on the MyPlate graphic.

One important change as you get older is that your calorie needs typically decrease after age 50; men generally need 2,000 daily calories and women 1,600, depending on physical activity. But your vitamin and mineral requirements stay the same or may even increase—which can make it a challenge to get the nutrients you need from a smaller calorie intake.

So, MyPlate for Older Adults provides examples of foods that contain high levels of vitamins and minerals per serving. These choices are also consistent with the dietary guidelines, which recommend limiting foods high in trans and saturated fats, salt, and added sugars.

Dense with Nutrients

If you're consuming fewer calories, it's important to get as many nutrients from those calories as possible. MyPlate for Older Adults spotlights vegetables and fruits as nutrient-dense food choices that are convenient, affordable, and readily available. Half of MyPlate for Older Adults is made up of fruit and vegetable icons, which reflects the importance of eating several servings of fruits and vegetables per day in a range of colors.

Consuming a variety of produce with deep-colored flesh introduces a larger amount of plant-based chemicals, nutrients, and fiber into your diet. MyPlate for Older Adults also includes icons representing frozen, pre-peeled fresh, dried, and certain low-sodium, low-sugar canned options. That's because fruits and vegetables in those forms contain as many or more nutrients as fresh and they are easier to prepare, are more affordable, and have a longer shelf life—all important considerations for older consumers.

MyPlate for Older Adults also features whole, enriched, and fortified grains because they are high in fiber and other beneficial nutrients. Experts advise making at least half your grain choices whole grains.

Suggested protein sources include fish and lean meat as well as plant-based options, such as beans and tofu. For cooking and serving, the Tufts experts recommend vegetable oils and soft spreads (free of trans fats—check the label) as alternatives to foods high in animal fats because animal-based products, such as butter and lard, are higher in saturated fat.

Other icons represent regular physical activity, emphasize adequate fluid intake, and focus on seasoning with herbs and spices instead of salt.

The MyPlate for Older Adults illustrates:

- Bright-colored vegetables, such as carrots and broccoli
- Deep-colored fruit, such as berries and peaches
- Whole, enriched, and fortified grains and cereals, such as brown rice and 100-percent whole wheat bread
- Low- and non-fat dairy products, such as yogurt and low-lactose milk
- Canned beans and unsalted nuts, fish, poultry, lean meat, and tofu
- Liquid vegetable oils, soft spreads low in saturated and trans fat, and spices to replace salt
- Fluids such as water, soups, teas, and fat-free milk
- Physical activity, such as walking, resistance training, and light cleaning

What to Avoid

Watching sodium intake is important for older people, not only for heart health but also because of the danger high blood pressure presents to the brain. "Blood pressure tends to increase as we age, so it is especially important for older adults to monitor dietary salt and, for most of us, try to find ways to decrease intake," says Tufts' Alice Lichtenstein, DSc, director of Tufts' HNRCA Cardiovascular Nutrition Laboratory. You can also cut down on salt by choosing the low-sodium options of items such as canned vegetables, and draining and rinsing canned beans. Excess sodium intake is only one of the unhealthy habits you should avoid to help protect your aging brain. One 17-year study of more than 5,000 English adults found that those with the unhealthiest behaviors were nearly three times more likely to suffer impairments in thinking and twice as likely to have memory problems as those with the healthiest lifestyles.

The study looked at the associations between cognition and four behaviors known to have negative overall health effects:

- Smoking
- Low fruit and vegetable consumption, defined as eating fewer than two servings of fruits and vegetables per day
- Lack of physical activity
- Alcohol abstinence versus moderate alcohol consumption, defined as drinking between 1 and 14 alcoholic beverages per week.

Compared to those with no unhealthy behaviors, those with three or four bad habits at early midlife were 84 percent more likely to have poor cognitive function 17 years later. As participants got older, the association between unhealthy behaviors and poor cognitive function was even stronger—nearly double.

Skip the Char

Even a habit as seemingly benign as blasting your food with high heat might be bad for your brain. In a study published in 2015 in the *Journal of Alzheimer's Disease*, researchers reported that chemicals called advanced glycation end products (AGEs), formed when foods are cooked at high temperatures, may contribute to the risk of developing Alzheimer's. Scientists used dietary survey data on the consumption of various foods to calculate that diets containing larger quantities of AGEs—especially from meats—correlated with higher incidence of Alzheimer's.

The study could only estimate AGE content, however, based on typical food preparations and the tendency of AGEs to form in certain foods. Researchers cautioned that other mechanisms could be responsible for the association, such as the fact that meat is also a source of saturated fat, which contributes to unhealthy cholesterol levels. To be on the safe side, turn down the temperature, avoid charring, and opt more often for braising meats in liquid.

Watch Your Weight

Being overweight or obese, not surprisingly, is another danger to your brain. A growing body of research links excess weight—also an important risk factor for heart disease—to cognitive decline and dementia.

To determine whether you're at risk, you can calculate your body mass index (BMI); this common measure compares your weight to your height. Some research has shown that the ratio of your waist to your hip measurement may be a more accurate measure of cardiovascular risk, although this hasn't been well tested for similar cognitive risks. Simply measuring your waistline, as if choosing the right pants size, also is a good general rule suggested by the American Heart Association and National Heart, Lung, and Blood Institute: Men should aim for a waist size less than 40 inches; women, less than 35 inches.

Brain Gains from Losing Weight

On the other hand, losing weight—especially combined with additional exercise—can benefit your brain. One study tested the cognitive benefits of a weight-loss diet, an exercise program, and dieting plus exercise among 107 frail, obese older adults for one year. Compared to a control group, all three regimens generally improved cognitive performance, though results varied by test.

But the combination of diet plus exercise was associated with the greatest improvement in MMMSE scores, word-fluency testing, and two "trail-making" tests of visual attention and task switching. Exercise alone boosted MMMSE and word fluency scores about the same as when combined with dieting.

Calorie Restriction

Several studies have reported that actively cutting down on calories—not simply "watching your weight"—might also be an effective strategy against cognitive decline. One German study found a connection between a restricted-calorie diet and improved memory among participants divided into three groups: One aimed to reduce calorie intake by 30 percent, mostly by eating smaller portions; a second group kept calories the same while increasing intake of healthy fats by 20 percent; and a third, the control group, made no dietary changes. At the end of three months, the calorie-cutting group scored an average of 20 percent better in tests of memory performance; the other groups showed no change. Researchers theorized that the calorie-cutters, who lost four to seven pounds, might experience brain benefits from decreased insulin and inflammation.

In another study, researchers compared the calorie intakes of older people suffering mild cognitive impairment (MCI) with normal control subjects. Those consuming the most calories—more than 2,143 per day—were almost twice as likely to have MCI than

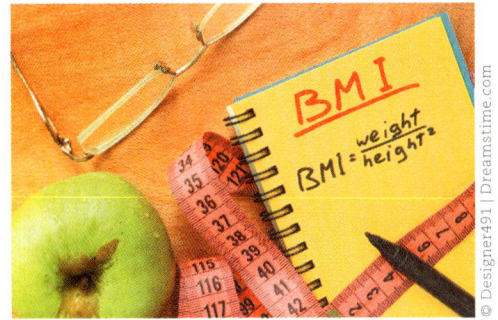

participants eating the least, fewer than 1,526 daily calories. The higher the amount of calories consumed each day, the higher the risk of MCI. The results were the same after adjusting for history of stroke, diabetes, amount of education, and other factors that can affect risk of memory loss.

Blood Sugar Risks

Being overweight or obese also affects your blood sugar levels, increasing the risk of diabetes. Chronically high blood-glucose (sugar) levels, whether from insulin resistance, prediabetes, or type 2 diabetes, seem in turn to affect the brain. One study linked higher blood glucose levels with a 40 percent greater risk of developing dementia. Blood glucose levels of diabetics who developed dementia over seven years averaged 190 mg/dl, compared to 160 mg/dl in those who did not develop dementia. (Normal fasting glucose levels are below 100 mg/dl and levels above 126 mg/dl are considered diabetes.)

People whose blood glucose is higher than normal but not high enough to meet the criteria for diabetes are also at greater risk. That same study found that people with the highest levels—but short of diabetes—were 20 percent more likely to develop dementia than those with normal blood-glucose levels. Among non-diabetic participants, those who developed dementia had blood-sugar levels averaging 115 mg/dl, compared with 109 mg/dl for those who did not develop dementia.

Hold the Starch

Smart choices about carbohydrates—another aspect of a healthy dietary pattern—can reduce your diabetes risk and help control your blood sugar. Recently, a large observational study linked starch consumption to greater risk of type 2 diabetes in women. Foods with a higher ratio of starch to fiber include processed and refined grain products, such as white rice, crackers, many ready-to-eat breakfast cereals, and bread and pasta that's not made from whole grains. Some vegetables, such as white potatoes and corn, are also high in starch. Intakes of total fiber, cereal fiber, and fruit fiber were all associated with lower diabetes risk.

FUNDAMENTAL NUTRIENTS

Fats, Carbohydrates, and Protein

You hear a lot about "nutrients," by which people typically mean vitamins, minerals, or even less-well-known nutrients such as flavonoids. The fundamental nutrients, however, are the familiar fats, carbohydrates, and protein. These are so basic to the nutritional quality of the foods we eat that their relative proportions are actually used to calculate how many calories are in a food. Rather than measure calories by literally burning up a food, most food manufacturers simply do the math: Fats have nine calories per gram, while carbohydrates and protein contain four calories. (When fiber, a form of carbohydrate, passes through the body without being digested, its calories don't "count.")

Total Fat Doesn't Count

The message that not all fat is bad for you hasn't gotten through to many people even today. All that worrying about the "Total Fat" line on the Nutrition Facts panel is a waste of time: Some types of fat—monounsaturated and polyunsaturated fats, like those found in liquid vegetable oils, nuts, and avocados—are actually good for your heart. That probably means they are also good for your brain. Fat is also an important component of cell membranes in the brain and of the myelin coating on neurons, which speeds up the transmission of information in the nervous system (see Box 3-1, "Fat Facts").

The latest Dietary Guidelines for Americans reversed 35 years of nutrition policy by omitting any recommended limit on total fat intake. In 1980, the federal Dietary Guidelines first recommended limiting dietary fat to less than 30 percent of calories; in a 2,000-calorie daily diet, that advice translated to a maximum of 65 grams of fat per day. The 1980 recommendation was revised in the 2005 guidelines to a range of 20 percent to 35 percent of calories from total fat. The percentages used in the Nutrition Facts panel, however, continue to be based on the 1980 recommendation of 30 percent or 65 grams.

Fats, Mediterranean Style

It's no coincidence that the Mediterranean-style diet, which seems to have cognitive benefits, is rich in healthy unsaturated fats. Scientists have found that increasing the intake of monounsaturated fats, as in olive oil, and of polyunsaturated fats, as in nuts, can help the brain perform its vital functions.

Participants in the PREDIMED-NAVARRA trial who followed a Mediterranean-style diet and also consumed at least four tablespoons of extra-virgin olive oil a day scored significantly better on two tests of mental abilities than a control group that was assigned to a low-fat diet. Those assigned to a Mediterranean plan supplemented with about a quarter-cup of walnuts, almonds, and hazelnuts daily

BOX 3-1

Fat Facts

Common sources of fats vary widely in their percentage of mono-, poly- and saturated fats:

	UNSATURATED		SATURATED
	MONO-	POLY-	
Canola oil	62%	32%	6%
Safflower oil	13%	77%	10%
Sunflower oil	20%	69%	11%
Corn oil	25%	62%	13%
Olive oil	77%	9%	14%
Soybean oil	24%	61%	15%
Peanut oil	49%	33%	18%
Lard	47%	12%	47%
Palm oil	39%	10%	51%
Butter	28%	4%	68%
Coconut oil	6%	2%	92%

Choose Healthy Fats and Fish for Your Brain

More evidence that polyunsaturated fats—including the omega-3 fats found in fish—have brain benefits comes from a large review of 21 observational studies totaling more than 180,000 participants. Researchers compared cognitive changes in middle-age and older adults for up to two decades with intakes of polyunsaturated fats and fish. Consuming an additional daily 8 grams of polyunsaturated fats was associated with a 29 percent lower risk of mild cognitive impairment and 10 percent lower risk of Parkinson's disease. Compared to not eating fish, consuming one serving per week of fish was associated with a 7 percent lower risk of Alzheimer's disease. Eating a weekly serving of fish was also associated with a 5 percent overall lower risk of dementia.

American Journal of Clinical Nutrition, February 2016

also scored better than the control group. After more than six-and-a-half years of follow-up, fewer participants consuming either of the Mediterranean-style diets were diagnosed with dementia than individuals in the control group.

The two Mediterranean groups actually consumed more total fat than the controls—but the fat was primarily heart-healthy monounsaturated (olive oil) or polyunsaturated (nuts). This finding further supports the apparent brain benefits of switching fats, rather than cutting down on fats of all types.

Go Unsaturated

In another study, scientists compared adherence to a Mediterranean-style eating pattern to white matter hyper-intensity volume (WMHV), a marker for small-blood-vessel damage in the brain. Participants completed food-frequency questionnaires to assess their diets and underwent MRI scans of their brains.

After adjustment for other risk factors, only one component of the Mediterranean diet was independently associated with WMHV: The ratio of monounsaturated fat to saturated fat. As the dietary share of monounsaturated fat rose versus saturated fat, WMHV declined. That suggests, researchers concluded, the overall dietary pattern rather than individual nutrients is responsible for healthier brains.

Butter and Other Saturated Fat: Still Don'ts

A few recent studies—and popular headlines—have cast doubt on the association between saturated fat and unhealthy cholesterol levels, some even proclaiming that "butter is back." Tufts experts, however, say, "Not so fast."

"We have strong data that substituting polyunsaturated fats for saturated fats decreases the risk of heart disease," says Tufts cardio-vascular nutrition expert Alice H. Lichtenstein. She adds, "We also have strong data that substituting carbohydrates, particularly refined carbohydrates, for saturated fats does not reduce risk." When data from studies that examine the effects of substituting polyunsaturated fats are analyzed together with those substituting carbohydrates for saturated fats, she says, the results can cause confusion.

Saturated Fat and Your Brain

What about cognitive effects? A recent review of the science published in *Neurobiology of Aging* generally supported a link between saturated fat intake and risk of Alzheimer's and dementia. Although some findings were mixed, saturated-fat intake was positively associated with Alzheimer's risk in three of four cohort studies. The review also found a positive association between saturated-fat intake and risk of dementia (one of two studies reviewed), risk of cognitive decline (two of four studies), and risk of mild cognitive impairment (one of two).

Previously, findings from the Women's Health Study showed that women who ate the most saturated fat had poorer scores on cognitive

BOX 3-3

tests than those who consumed the least and were about 65 percent more likely to experience a decline in mental performance over time. The total amount of fat intake did not really matter, but the type of fat did.

Keys to Cholesterol

Along with trans fat, saturated fat is believed to contribute to unhealthy cholesterol in your bloodstream, called "serum" cholesterol. That cholesterol—a waxy, fat-like substance—is not the same as the dietary cholesterol listed on Nutrition Facts panels. The latest expert guidance largely dismisses concerns over intake of dietary cholesterol, such as that found in eggs and shellfish.

Your body needs a little serum cholesterol. But your body can make all the cholesterol it needs, primarily in the liver; any extra cholesterol can get deposited in artery walls.

Atherosclerosis Risks

This accumulated cholesterol eventually forms plaque, which narrows blood vessels and makes them less flexible—resulting in atherosclerosis, popularly known as "hardening of the arteries." Since your brain uses such a high proportion of your body's blood flow, anything that affects your circulation also impacts your brain (see Box 3-3, "Cholesterol Process").

The Diabetes Heart Study-Mind found that such changes in the vascular system were related to cognition even before the changes became clinically apparent and treatable. Researchers measured the amount of calcified plaque in participants' coronary arteries when the study began. Seven years later, a battery of cognitive tests measured subjects' memory, processing speed, and executive function: Those with greater plaque at baseline scored lower on those mental tests.

Your Cholesterol Numbers

Just as oil and water don't mix, fatty serum cholesterol and watery blood can't directly combine. So, cholesterol in your blood rides along in packages called lipoproteins, which have cholesterol inside and protein on the outside. The two main types of these lipoproteins are what are actually measured when the lab tests your cholesterol. Here is what those numbers mean:

- **Low-density lipoprotein, or LDL,** is known as "bad" cholesterol because it carries cholesterol to your tissues. When too much LDL circulates in the blood, it can slowly build up in the walls of the arteries that supply blood to the heart and brain. According to the American Heart Association, an LDL cholesterol level of 130 to 159 mg/dL (milligrams per deciliter) is "borderline high," 160 to 189 mg/dL is "high," and 190 mg/dL and above is "very high."
- **High-density lipoprotein, or HDL,** carries cholesterol from tissues to the liver, which removes it from the body; this earns it the nickname of "good" cholesterol. A level of at least 40 mg/dL for men and

Cholesterol Process

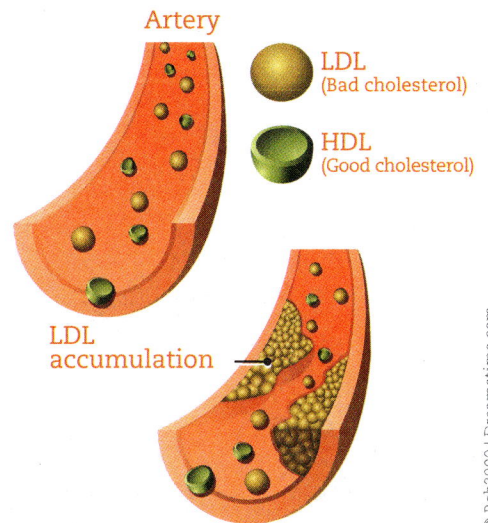

© Rob3000 | Dreamstime.com

HDL, the "good" cholesterol, transports LDL, the "bad" cholesterol, out of the cells that line arterial walls, which reduces the amount of plaque in the arteries and permits better blood flow, as well as reducing the risk of cardiovascular events.

50 mg/dL for women is associated with lower risk; the higher the HDL, the better.

♦ **Triglycerides are another form of fat in your blood.** Calories you consume that are not used immediately by the body's tissues are converted to triglycerides and transported to fat cells to be stored. Hormones regulate the release of triglycerides from fat tissue to meet the body's energy needs between meals. An excess of triglycerides in the blood, a condition called hypertriglyceridemia, is linked to the occurrence of coronary artery disease in some people. According to the American Heart Association, a triglyceride level of 150 to 199 mg/dL is "borderline high," 200 to 499 mg/dL is "high," and 500 mg/dL and above is "very high."

Statins Plus Diet

For most people, statin medications are powerfully effective for reducing cholesterol. levels But you can also improve unhealthy cholesterol levels by adjusting your diet. To reduce LDL cholesterol, the American Heart Association recommends limiting saturated-fat intake to five to six percent of your total calories (see Box 3-4 "Fat Content of Common Foods"). For most people, this means cutting saturated-fat intake roughly in half; the current average intake is 11 percent of calories. In a 2,000-calories daily diet, five to six percent of calories would equal 100 to 120 calories a day from saturated fat. That translates to roughly 11 to 13 grams of saturated fat per day, or a little less than the saturated fat in two tablespoons of butter or a five-ounce serving of rib-eye steak.

It's key to replace those unhealthy fats with healthy ones—not, as in the fat-free fad of recent years, with refined carbohydrates. For best results, experts advise, substitute polyunsaturated fat for saturated fat. Next best is monounsaturated fat.

You also should avoid trans fats, found in partially hydrogenated oils used in some baked goods and packaged products. Both saturated fats and trans fats raise LDL; trans fats also lower healthy HDL.

BOX 3-4

Fat Content of Common Foods

FOOD AND SERVING SIZE	SATURATED FAT	MONOUNSATURATED FAT	POLYUNSATURATED FAT	TRANS FAT
Egg, 1 large	1.6g	1.8g	1g	<0.1g
85% lean ground beef, 1/4-lb patty	4.5g	5.1g	0.3g	0.4g
Chicken breast, boneless, skinless, 4oz	1.1g	1.6g	0.9g	<0.1g
Strip steak, 4 oz	9.5g	10.3g	1g	0.1g
Glazed cruller doughnut, 3" dia.	1.9g	4.3g	0.9g	n/a
Pepperoni pizza, 1 slice	5.7g	4.3g	2.3g	0.3g
Fries, fast-food medium	2.7g	8.6g	5.5g	<0.1g
American cheese, 1 slice (1 oz)	5.1g	2.3g	0.4g	0.3g
Macaroni and cheese, 1 cup	3.1g	4.2g	2g	0.2g
Vanilla ice cream, regular fat, ½ cup	4.5g	2.1g	0.3g	n/a
Latte made with 2% milk, 16 oz.	4.5g	2.0g	0.5g	<0.1g

HDL and Cognition

Scientists continue to investigate the role of that "good" cholesterol in your body. Some studies have failed to find benefits from boosting HDL cholesterol, suggesting that this number may actually be just a marker for an overall healthy lifestyle.

On the other hand, a study of 3,673 men and women suggests that higher HDL cholesterol might benefit the brain. Researchers measured cholesterol levels twice, at average ages 55 and 61, and short-term verbal memory was tested at each age. Initially, participants with low HDL (less than 40 mg/dL) scored lower on the memory test than those with high HDL (60 mg/dL or higher), but the difference wasn't statistically significant. After five years, however, the difference increased to become significant. Moreover, individuals whose HDL levels declined during the five-year interval were more likely to also show a decline in memory performance than those whose HDL levels did not change.

The researchers speculated that HDL might protect cognitive function by reducing the risk for stroke and vascular disease, or HDL could moderate beta-amyloid, which is associated with plaques in the brain. Additionally, HDL may have anti-inflammatory or antioxidant effects, which could help to prevent the degeneration of the brain's neurons.

You can maintain healthy HDL levels by not smoking, avoiding trans fats, and losing weight. Factors thought to boost HDL include exercise, moderate alcohol consumption, and intake of soluble dietary fiber, such as that found in oats, vegetables, fruits, and legumes.

Inflammation and Chronic Disease

Inflammation is part of your body's natural defense mechanism, but chronic inflammation in the blood vessels can allow LDL cholesterol to invade, producing a vicious circle of increasing inflammation. Markers of inflammation in the bloodstream also have been linked to cognitive decline and abnormalities in brain structure. As people age, the regulatory processes that combat inflammation become less effective, resulting in greater inflammatory responses and damage.

Systemic inflammation is associated with a range of chronic diseases that are also related to diet, obesity, and lack of physical activity—notably cardiovascular disease and type 2 diabetes. Fat (adipose) tissue is a source of chemicals that promote inflammation. Many risk factors for decline in brain health—including free radicals (countered by antioxidants) and homocysteine (related to B vitamins)—can trigger inflammatory responses in the brain. And so can oxidized lipids, related to unhealthy cholesterol levels.

The best strategy for combating inflammation is to make the healthy lifestyle changes that can reduce your risk of chronic disease. We'll look at these risk factors in-depth in later chapters (see Box 3-5, "Inflammation").

BOX 3-5

Inflammation

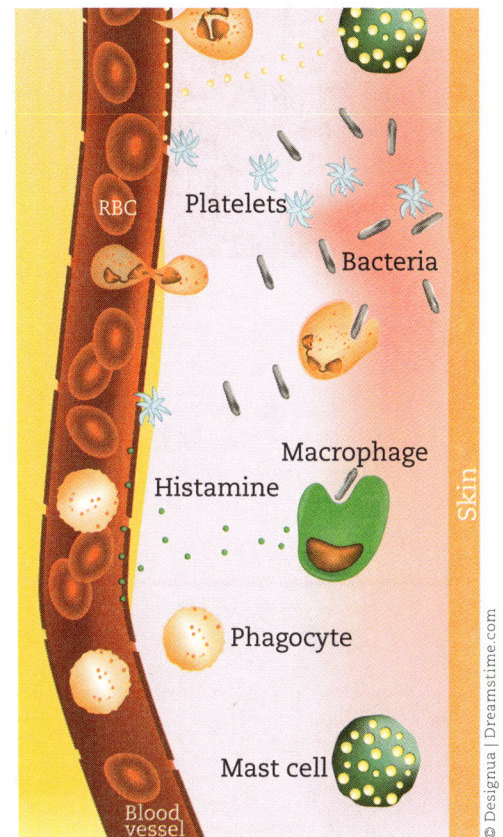

Inflammation is part of the body's immune response, the process by which the body responds to injury or infection. During this process, damaged tissues release histamines, which increase blood flow to the area. Histamines cause capillaries to leak, releasing phagocytes that rid the body of bacteria, dead cells, and cellular debris. During chronic inflammation, however, the body can turn on itself, damaging healthy tissue and causing autoimmune diseases, such as rheumatoid arthritis. Research suggests that chronic inflammation can restrict blood flow to both the heart and brain, and it has been implicated as a major risk factor in both heart disease and dementia.

Omega-6s and Inflammation

Another common type of fatty acid is called omega-6, found in liquid vegetable oils high in polyunsaturated fats, including corn, safflower, sunflower, and soybean oils, as well as walnuts and soybeans. Linoleic acid (LA) is the essential omega-6 fatty acid, meaning the body can't produce it but must obtain it from dietary sources; LA is necessary for normal growth, development, and brain function. But you may have seen warnings, on the Internet or in popular nutrition books, about the dangers of omega-6 fatty acids, which supposedly cause inflammation. Some experts have recommended lowering the ratio of omega-6 fats to omega-3 fats to combat this risk.

It's true that some of the main omega-6 fatty acids are involved in the early stages of inflammation, but they also give rise to *anti-inflammatory* molecules. A recent American Heart Association review, however, concluded that higher intakes of omega-6s "appear to be safe and may be even more beneficial (as part of a low–saturated-fat, low-cholesterol diet)."

In fact, an analysis published in *Circulation* found that people who swap 5 percent of the calories they consume from saturated fat sources, such as red meat and butter, with foods containing linoleic acid saw a 9 percent lower risk of coronary heart disease events. Switching from saturated fat to linoleic acid was also associated with a 13 percent lower coronary heart disease mortality risk. Since what's good for the heart is good for the brain, this suggests there's no reason to fear omega-6 fats.

Carbs: Fiber, Sugar, and Starch

After the "fat-free" craze, the next target for a healthy-eating fad was carbohydrates. Going "low-carb," it was claimed, would lead to dramatic weight loss and other health benefits. In extreme forms, this fad meant cutting back even on healthy sources of carbohydrates, such as fruits and vegetables.

Not surprisingly, the reality about the health effects of carbohydrates is more complicated than such fads take into account. Carbohydrates—composed of sugars, starches, and fiber—provide energy for the body, especially the brain and the nervous system. To obtain that energy, enzymes break down carbohydrates into glucose (blood sugar) during digestion, which the body then uses to fuel its many functions.

So, your brain needs some carbohydrates, and it suffers when you don't get enough. Dietary fiber, a type of carbohydrate that passes through your body undigested, has beneficial effects on your cardiovascular system that can in turn help protect your brain. (When counting "net" carbohydrates, subtract fiber from the total, since it doesn't get digested like sugar and starch.) Sugar, however, especially in the form of added sugar that comes with no extra vitamins or minerals (versus, for example, the sugar in a piece of fruit), is increasingly seen as a key contributor to chronic disease. And research is beginning to implicate starch, such as that in refined grain products, as an important culprit in weight gain and diabetes.

Carbohydrate Math

You can quickly see the fiber and sugar content of foods on the Nutrition Facts panel, and recent pending revisions to the panel include a separate

BOX 3-6

listing of added sugars (see Box 3-6, "Old vs. New Nutrition Facts Labels"). To find the starch content takes just a bit of math: Subtract the fiber and sugar grams from the total grams of carbohydrates. To calculate the starch content of a one-cup serving of corn flakes, for example, subtract the fiber (1) and sugar (3) grams from the total carbohydrates (24): 24-1-3=20 grams of starch (about the same amount as in a cup of potatoes).

Simple vs. Complex

Carbohydrates are also classified as simple or complex—a distinction that confuses many people. Simple carbohydrates are made up of one (single) or two (double) sugar molecules. When most people think of simple carbohydrates, they think of sucrose (a double sugar), the stuff you sprinkle on cereal or spoon into your coffee. But that's only the most familiar simple carbohydrate. Others include glucose (a single sugar found in most fruits), fructose (a single sugar also found in fruits), galactose (a single sugar found in dairy products), lactose (a double sugar found in dairy products), and maltose (found in certain vegetables and in beer).

The nutritional value of simple carbohydrates depends on the foods in which they are found—they are not necessarily bad for you or to be avoided just because they're "simple." The simple sugars, such as those found in candy, non-diet sodas, syrups, and table sugar, provide calories, but few other nutrients. In contrast, intake of nutritious foods, such as fruits, vegetables, milk, and other dairy products, provides not only calories from sugar, but also essential vitamins and minerals.

Starch Cautions

Carbohydrates that have three or more sugars are called complex. These "starchy" carbohydrates are found in foods including beans and other legumes, starchy vegetables (corn, potatoes), and whole-grain breads and cereals. The health impact of complex carbohydrates, again, depends on what else they bring to the table. Legumes, vegetables, and whole grains provide essential nutrients; on the other hand, refined complex carbohydrates, such as white flour, are stripped of many of their original nutrients in processing.

Doubts About the Glycemic Index

One reason starchy foods might contribute to weight gain and diabetes risk is that they tend to have a higher glycemic index (GI), a measure of how quickly your body converts a food to glucose. Low-GI foods are slowly digested and include lentils, soybeans, and many whole grains. In contrast, high-GI foods are converted to glucose more rapidly; these include potatoes and white bread.

When a food's typical serving size is factored along with its glycemic index, the result is called the glycemic load. Choosing lower-glycemic foods is generally associated with health benefits, including possible reduced risk of type 2 diabetes, though recent research has questioned the cardiovascular benefits of low-GI eating.

Old vs. New Nutrition Facts Labels

Nutrition Facts

Serving Size 2/3 cup (55g)
Servings Per Container About 8

Amount Per Serving

Calories 230	Calories from Fat 72

	% Daily Value*
Total Fat 8g	**12%**
Saturated Fat 1g	**5%**
Trans Fat 0g	
Cholesterol 0mg	**0%**
Sodium 160mg	**7%**
Total Carbohydrate 37g	**12%**
Dietary Fiber 4g	**16%**
Sugars 12g	
Protein 3g	

Vitamin A	10%
Vitamin C	8%
Calcium	20%
Iron	45%

* Percent Daily Values are based on a 2,000 calorie diet. Your daily value may be higher or lower depending on your calorie needs.

		Calories:	2,000	2,500
Total Fat	Less than		65g	80g
Sat Fat	Less than		20g	25g
Cholesterol	Less than		300mg	300mg
Sodium	Less than		2,400mg	2,400mg
Total Carbohydrate			300g	375g
Dietary Fiber			25g	30g

▲ Old Nutrition Label ▲

Nutrition Facts

8 servings per container
Serving size   2/3 cup (55g)

Amount per serving
Calories   230

	% Daily Value*
Total Fat 8g	**12%**
Saturated Fat 1g	**5%**
Trans Fat 0g	
Cholesterol 0mg	**0%**
Sodium 160mg	**7%**
Total Carbohydrate 37g	**12%**
Dietary Fiber 4g	**16%**
Total Sugars 12g	
Includes 10g Added Sugars	**20%**
Protein 3g	

Vitamin D 2mcg	10%
Calcium 260mg	20%
Iron 8mg	45%
Potassium 235mg	6%

* The % Daily Value (DV) tells you how much a nutrient in a serving of food contributes to a daily diet. 2,000 calories a day is used for general nutrition advice.

▲ New Nutrition Label ▲

FDA.gov/Food/GuidanceRegulation/GuidanceDocumentsRegulatoryInformation/LabelingNutrition

BOX 3-7

What Are Whole Grains?

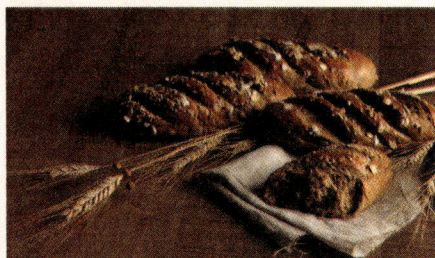

Whole grains, or foods made from them, contain all the essential parts and naturally occurring nutrients of the entire grain seed. If the grain has been processed—e.g., cracked, crushed, rolled, extruded, and/or cooked (but leaving the original kernel intact), the food product should deliver approximately the same rich balance of nutrients that are found in the original grain seed. This definition means that 100 percent of the original kernel—all the bran, germ, and endosperm—are present. Because whole grains are digested more slowly than processed carbohydrates, they have a less dramatic effect on blood sugar—and thus may be better for the brain.

These grains are examples of generally accepted whole-grain foods and flours:

- Amaranth
- Barley
- Buckwheat
- Corn, including whole cornmeal and popcorn
- Millet
- Oats, including oatmeal
- Quinoa
- Rice, both brown rice and colored rice
- Rye
- Sorghum (also called milo)
- Teff
- Triticale
- Wheat, including varieties such as spelt, emmer, farro, einkorn, Kamut, durum, and forms such as bulgur, cracked wheat, and wheatberries
- Wild rice

Whole Grains Council (wholegrainscouncil.org)

The evidence for brain benefits of a low-GI diet is also inconsistent. Some studies have shown benefits, while others failed to find any differences, and still other studies showed effects on only some aspects of cognitive performance.

Moreover, new Tufts research has questioned the utility of commonly used glycemic index values. According to 2016 findings published in the *American Journal of Clinical Nutrition*, actual blood-sugar effects can vary by an average of 20% within an individual and 25% among individuals. "Glycemic-index values appear to be an unreliable indicator even under highly standardized conditions and are unlikely to be useful in guiding food choices," says lead study author Nirupa Matthan, PhD, a scientist in the HNRCA Cardiovascular Nutrition Laboratory. "If someone eats the same amount of the same food three times, their blood-glucose response should be similar each time, but that was not observed in our study. A food that is low glycemic index for you one time you eat it could be high the next time, and it may have no impact on blood sugar for me."

Carbohydrate Conclusions

So what's the bottom line on carbohydrates and your brain? As with fats, carbohydrates are neither all good nor all bad. Tufts researchers have even found that very low-carbohydrate diets could have a negative impact on thinking and cognition. That's likely because the brain doesn't store glucose, its primary fuel, but depends on the body's production of it from carbohydrates in the diet. After only a day or two, even the glucose stored by the body is exhausted and must be replenished from the diet.

Other research has linked consumption of certain kinds of carbohydrates to possible brain benefits. An 11-year assessment of diet and cognitive function among nearly 4,000 older men and women found: "Whole grains and nuts and legumes were positively associated with higher cognitive functions and may be core neuroprotective foods common to various healthy plant-centered diets around the globe" (See Box 3-7, "What Are Whole Grains?").

On the other hand, consuming too many carbohydrates relative to protein and fat seems to contribute to cognitive decline. In one study, scientists reported that people 70 and older who ate the highest proportion of carbohydrates were at nearly four times the risk of developing mild cognitive impairment than their counterparts who ate relatively fewer carbohydrates. Risk also rose with a diet heavy in sugar. Study participants who consumed more protein and fat relative to carbohydrates were less likely to become cognitively impaired.

Protein Power

Despite the booming popularity of protein on supermarket shelves, most Americans probably already get plenty of protein—and too many of the calories and saturated fats that accompany animal sources of protein. The Daily Value (DV) for protein used on the Nutrition Facts panel percentages is 50 grams. Most of us far exceed that number, with actual consumption estimated at 62 to 66 grams of protein daily for women and 88 to 92 grams for men (see Box 3-8, "Your Protein Plan").

The protein equation may be different for older people, however. "It's estimated that 20 percent of people between the ages of 51 and 70 have an inadequate protein intake," says Paul Jacques, DSc, director of Tufts' HNRCA Nutritional Epidemiology Program. Often, older people simply eat less as appetites wane, and that means consuming less protein.

Recent research by Dr. Jacques and colleagues, in fact, found that to get the most out of exercise, older participants also had to be consuming enough protein. Participants who did muscle-strengthening exercises without protein intake of at least 70 grams daily actually had *lower* muscle mass.

Protein for Breakfast

How much protein you need really depends on your body weight—0.8 grams of protein per 2.2 pounds. For example, a 125-pound woman would need 46 grams of protein per day, while a 175-pound man would need 64 grams per day. If you are very physically active, you may need to increase that. You might also want to spread your protein consumption through the day, rather than concentrating it at dinnertime (see Box 3-9, "Timing Your Protein").

When you eat your daily protein may be as important as how much you consume, Dr. Jacques adds: "Meeting a protein threshold of approximately 25 to 30 grams per meal represents a promising yet relatively unexplored dietary strategy to help maintain muscle mass and function in older adults." Breakfast, he says, may provide the greatest opportunity to more evenly distribute the day's protein.

As you age, protein is essential to prevent the loss of lean muscle mass, called "sarcopenia," and for the brain. Protein is important to your brain for the production of neurotransmitters and enzymes, and to maintain the structural components of the brain.

So you should aim to consume enough protein from lean, healthy sources to keep your muscles and brain strong, while avoiding the extra calories and saturated fats that accompany less-healthy protein sources.

Balancing Act

The changing recommendations of how best to balance fats, carbohydrates, and proteins in a brain-healthy diet can seem like a roller coaster. That "roller coaster" is best understood as not a circular ride at all, however, but an occasionally winding journey. As science uncovers new evidence, naturally, those dietary recommendations will detour to match. That's the nature of science and discovery—otherwise, our maps would still warn, "Here there be dragons."

The best advice is to use your brain—in the form of common sense—to eat right to protect it. Avoid fad diets, quick fixes, and radical swings to extremes, while embracing the healthy choices we'll explore in-depth in the next chapter.

BOX 3-8

Your Protein Plan

Make sure that you're consuming high-quality protein, containing all the essential amino acids your body must obtain from dietary sources. Grains (with the notable exception of quinoa) are usually not an adequate source of the amino acids lysine and isoleucine. Legumes, such as beans, tend to fall short in delivering a different amino acid, methionine. (This is why eating a grain like rice together with beans is a good idea, to obtain a complete range of amino acids.) Meat, poultry, fish, eggs, dairy products, and soy are all sources of complete proteins.

BOX 3-9

Timing Your Protein

You may want to spread your protein consumption through the day, rather than concentrating it at dinner time; changing body chemistry means older adults benefit from a more even distribution of protein intake. Some experts recommend that seniors consume 25 to 30 grams of high-quality protein with each meal to maximize the body's synthesis of muscle protein. That's a lot more protein than you'll get from a typical breakfast of cereal and juice, which delivers only about eight grams. Consider adding an egg, low-fat cottage cheese, whole-wheat toast, meatless breakfast sausage, or even fish to your breakfast to make sure your body has plenty of protein to start the day.

FEEDING YOUR BRAIN

While the most important nutritional protection you can give your brain involves eating an overall healthy dietary pattern, it's also true that certain specific foods and food groups seem to be especially important for brain health (see Box 4-1, "Brain Food"). Fortunately, these brain-healthy choices are also good for your cardiovascular system and overall health. So, as you feed your brain, you'll also be taking care of the rest of your body.

The Positives of Fruits and Vegetables

It's no surprise that fruits and vegetables play a dominant role in brain-healthy patterns of eating, just as they do in healthy diets for your body as a whole (see Box 4-2, "How Much Produce Is Enough?"). But, it may be that eating fruits and vegetables helps protect your brain beyond general health benefits.

Berries for Your Brain

As we saw with the MIND diet in chapter 2, research on the brain benefits of specific foods has focused in particular on berries. Pigment compounds called anthocyanins that give berries their distinctive red, purple, and blue colors can cross the blood-brain barrier to become localized in areas of the brain related to learning and memory. Anthocyanins are found in fruits such as blueberries, strawberries, raspberries, blackberries, bilberries, huckleberries, and cranberries, as well as grapes and currants. In the brain, anthocyanins decrease vulnerability to the oxidative stress that occurs with aging, reduce inflammation, and may increase neuronal signaling.

Recent research in animals at Tufts further bolsters evidence for the potential brain benefits of berries. Barbara Shukitt-Hale, PhD, and her colleagues tested blueberry and strawberry powders added to the diets of 42 aged lab rats. Compared to rats fed only their normal chow, those consuming diets supplemented with berries had enhanced motor performance and improved cognition, specifically working memory. The berries also boosted production of neurons in the hippocampus and of insulin-like growth factor 1 (ILGF 1), which has been associated with learning and memory. The different polyphenol compounds in the berries also produced some different results: Rats getting blueberry powder performed better on psychomotor coordination, for example, while those in the strawberry group did better in tests of general balance and coordination.

Previous animal studies conducted at Tufts found that the addition of blueberries to the diet improved short-term memory, navigational skills, balance, coordination, and reaction time. Compounds in blueberries seem to jump-start the brain in ways that get aging neurons to communicate again.

Berries Beyond the Lab

Evidence for a similar benefit in humans comes from an analysis of data on berry consumption among some 16,000 women over age 70

BOX 4-2

How Much Produce Is Enough?

The USDA's MyPlate calls for filling half your plate with fruits and vegetables, and recommends that people over age 50 consume one-and-a-half to two cups daily of fruit and two to two-and-a-half cups of vegetables. For less-dense produce, such as salad greens, count two cups as the equivalent of one cup of other vegetables.

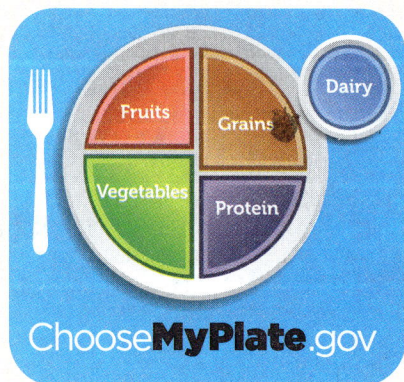

BOX 4-1

Brain Food

The science of whether some dietary choices are really "brain food" continues to unfold. Given the long time frames of conditions such as Alzheimer's disease and other dementias, it's challenging to prove any cause and effect relationship between specific foods and brain health. Most such associations are drawn from observational studies, in which people who eat more or less of a certain food are assessed over time for cognitive changes. It's obviously difficult to feed a group of study participants lots of, say, blueberries for several years in order to test their brain health at the end; that's why clinical trials of foods and the brain have largely depended on animal tests.

Nonetheless, some foods tend to stand out from the pages and pages of research results as most likely being protective for brain health. These "brain foods" typically contain one or more nutrients that scientists believe have positive effects on the brain and/or the cardiovascular system, which in turn affects the brain. These foods include:

- **Berries,** such as blueberries, strawberries, raspberries, blackberries, bilberries, huckleberries, cranberries, and açai berries, all of which contain anthocyanins that combat free radicals and oxidative stress. Blueberries in particular are important in the MIND diet.

- **Other deeply colored, berry-like fruits,** including grapes and currants. These fruits also contain resveratrol, which is being studied for its health effects.

- **Vegetables,** especially those high in vitamin E, such as spinach, kale, and other leafy greens, avocados, broccoli, and asparagus. Eating more vegetables is, of course, good for your overall health, and people who eat more vegetables are less prone to cognitive decline.

- **Nuts of all kinds,** including peanuts (technically legumes). These nutritional powerhouses, high in vitamin E and magnesium, are packed with healthy unsaturated fats and have proven cardiovascular benefits.

- **Dark chocolate and cocoa** contain phytochemical compounds called flavanols that have also been shown to have cardiovascular benefits. Recent studies have similarly found associations between chocolate consumption and benefits for memory and other aspects of cognition.

- **Coffee** has been shown to help protect the arteries, which is one way in which coffee consumption could also be good for the brain. Coffee also contains caffeine, which not only stimulates the brain in the short term but may protect against long-term cognitive decline later in life.

- **Tea,** especially green tea, contains phytochemicals that seem to benefit working memory and may help counter the plaques that characterize Alzheimer's disease. Tea, as well as herbal teas containing hibiscus, also has been found to help control high blood pressure, which is the number-one risk factor for brain-damaging strokes and vascular dementia.

- **Seafood,** especially varieties of fish high in heart-healthy omega-3 fatty acids, such as salmon, trout, sardines, herring, and mackerel, protects the brain by its cardiovascular benefits and may also have direct brain benefits. DHA, one of the two primary omega-3s

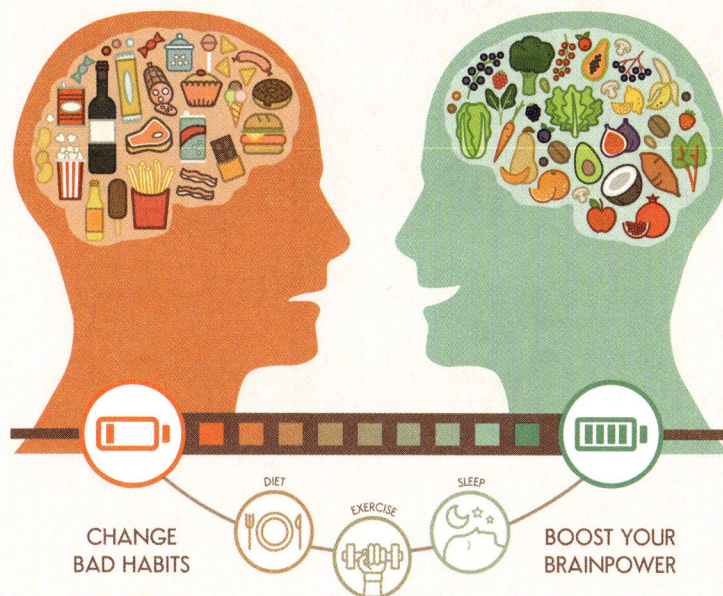

CHANGE BAD HABITS — DIET — EXERCISE — SLEEP — BOOST YOUR BRAINPOWER

© Elenabsl | Dreamstime.com

in fish oil, is a key component in brain development and the most important fatty acid in the brain. People at higher genetic risk of Alzheimer's may particularly benefit from eating more fish. Other studies have suggested that older people see greater cognitive benefits from fish consumption than those in midlife.

Part of a Pattern

These foods are most effective when consumed as part of an overall healthy dietary pattern—you can't just eat a few blueberries to make up for the deleterious effects of gorging on pizza and cheeseburgers. Tufts' MyPlate for Older Adults recommends a plate "makeover" at your meals, so that your dietary intake includes:

- 50% fruits and vegetables
- 25% grains, most of which are whole grains; and
- 25% protein-rich foods, such as nuts, beans, fish, lean meat, poultry, and fat-free and low-fat dairy products, such as milk, cheeses, and yogurts.

The plan also calls for plenty of healthy sources of fluids, such as water, milk, tea, soup, and coffee. You should choose heart-healthy monounsaturated and polyunsaturated fats such as vegetable oils and soft margarines, limiting intake of saturated fats from animal products, such as butter, lard, and fatty red and processed meats. Tufts experts also advise using herbs and spices in place of salt to lower sodium intake, which contributes to high blood pressure.

A brain-healthy diet should also limit intake of added sugars, which don't come with any compensating nutrients, and of refined grains and starchy foods.

As you age, be aware that you may not be getting enough of certain nutrients important to your body and brain, because of reduced intake, impaired absorption, or medications. These include vitamin B12, vitamin D, calcium, iron, zinc, and dietary fiber. It's also important to drink plenty of water and other non-caloric fluids, as your sensitivity to thirst may decline with age.

Other healthy dietary plans that contain plenty of "brain food" include the Mediterranean diet, the Dietary Approaches to Stop Hypertension (DASH) plan, and the MIND diet, discussed in chapter 2.

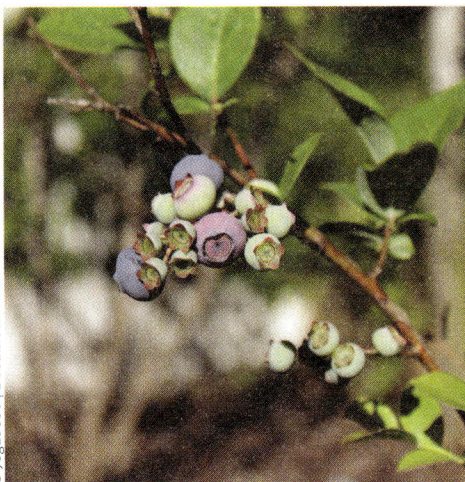

Berries, such as blueberries, retain their healthy qualities when dried or frozen and can be enjoyed year round.

participating in the Nurses' Health Study. The women were tested for memory and other cognitive functions every two years and completed dietary questionnaires every four years. Researchers found that those who consumed two or more half-cup servings of strawberries or blueberries per week experienced slower mental decline—equivalent over time to up to two and a half years of delayed aging.

In other research, some data in Alzheimer's patients indicate that blueberries could forestall the brain damage that is a hallmark of the disease.

Berries, such as blueberries, retain their healthy qualities when dried or frozen and can be enjoyed year round. Consider starting your day with a smoothie that contains a few handfuls of blueberries (using frozen berries reduces the amount of ice you need to add to your blender).

While whole fruits (even pureed in a blender) are a healthier choice than juices, which sacrifice most of the fruits' fiber content, the anthocyanins in berries and grapes seem to survive juicing. Randomized controlled trials have produced promising evidence for the effects of cranberry, blueberry, and grape juice on cognitive performance in older adults.

One study, for example, tested the effects of Concord grape juice versus a placebo beverage in elderly volunteers, who were already suffering mild cognitive impairment. After 16 weeks, those who drank grape juice scored better on tests of memory than those in the placebo group. Measurement of brain activity using functional magnetic resonance imaging revealed greater activation in key parts of the brain among the grape-juice group, suggesting increased blood flow in areas of the brain associated with learning and memory.

Phytochemicals Feed Your Brain

The anthocyanins in berries and the compounds called polyphenols found in apple, grape, and citrus fruits and juices (particularly those that have been mechanically squeezed with the peels) are examples of natural plant compounds called phytochemicals (or phytonutrients). Diane L. McKay, PhD, an assistant professor at the Tufts' Friedman School and a scientist in its Human Nutrition Research Center on Aging Antioxidants Laboratory, explains, "These are not classic nutrients like vitamins. These are compounds present in plants that have biological activity that confers health benefits, such as improving markers of disease risk. All phytochemicals have antioxidant activity, but that is not necessarily their mode of action in the body

There is growing evidence that fruits and vegetables containing phytochemicals can counteract age-related declines in cognitive functioning. Among the most-studied phytochemicals are the large group of polyphenols, which include catechins (found, for example, in tea) and flavanols (found in chocolate).

For a Youthful Brain, Eat Your Veggies

Eating more vegetables also has been associated with cognitive protection. One study at Rush University found that two servings a day of vegetables prevented the equivalent of five years of mental aging. Participants who ate at least 2.8 servings of vegetables a day over a span of six years slowed their rate of cognitive decline as measured by standardized tests by about 40 percent compared to those who consumed less than one serving a day. Researchers speculated that the high vitamin E content of vegetables might be key to this apparent benefit, noting that vegetables are typically consumed with some fats, which increases the absorption of vitamin E and other fat-soluble antioxidant nutrients.

Another study, involving nearly 2,000 older, dementia-free Japanese-Americans, provides support for the idea that vegetable juice as well as whole vegetables may help fend off Alzheimer's disease. In the nine-year study, participants who drank at least three glasses of fruit or vegetable juice per week were 76 percent less likely to develop Alzheimer's compared with those who averaged less than one glass per week. Even those who drank only one or two servings weekly had some protection compared with those who consumed less juice.

Nuts Not Just an Indulgence

Once thought of as an indulgence, nuts are increasingly being recognized as a contributor to an overall healthy diet. Consuming nuts can help improve cholesterol levels and protect your heart and arteries, which is also good for your brain. Some studies also have looked specifically at possible cognitive benefits from nuts (see Box 4-3, "Almonds Counter Post-Lunch Brain Dip").

In the Spanish PREDIMED study, adding extra nuts to the Mediterranean diet seemed to boost protection for aging brains. Those consuming a Mediterranean diet plus an ounce of mixed nuts daily scored better in tests of memory than participants assigned to a control group.

In a study done at Tufts, the phytochemicals and healthy fats in walnuts seemed to improve brain function in laboratory rats. For eight weeks, the animals were randomly assigned to eat a diet containing zero percent, two percent, six percent, or nine percent walnuts. Then, they were given age-sensitive tests of balance, coordination, and spatial memory. Rats that consumed the two percent and six percent walnut-enriched diets showed improved motor and cognitive function. The six-percent-walnut diet would equate to a human eating one ounce of nuts per day. Intake of larger amounts of walnuts did not provide additional benefits.

Nut Nutrition

Like other plant foods, nuts—including not only tree nuts but also peanuts (technically legumes)—are rich sources of phytochemicals. These little nutritional powerhouses are also excellent sources of vitamin E and magnesium. Individuals consuming nuts have higher intakes of folate, beta-carotene, vitamin K, lutein plus zeaxanthin, phosphorus, copper, selenium, potassium, and zinc than those who do not consume nuts.

Though nuts vary in their mix of vitamins, minerals, and heart-healthy fats, the type of nut you choose to consume probably doesn't matter much. You might do best by simply eating a variety of nuts, consumed as a substitute for less-healthy snacks.

NEW FINDING   BOX 4-3

Almonds Counter Post-Lunch Brain Dip

Brain fading a bit after lunch? Try a handful of almonds. The "post-lunch dip" in cognition is a well-established phenomenon of decreased alertness, memory, and vigilance; dieters are particularly prone to cognitive function impairments. A new study set out to test the cognitive effects of an almond-enriched lunch, rich in healthy unsaturated fats, versus a high-carbohydrate lunch, as part of a 12-week weight-loss intervention. The 86 overweight and obese adults were randomly assigned to either an almond-enhanced diet (55 percent of calories from fat, 70 to 75 percent of calories from almonds) or a lunch with 85 percent of calories coming from carbohydrates, at the beginning and end of the weight-loss program. Measures of memory and attention did drop after lunch, as expected. But the almond-enriched high-fat lunch ameliorated the post-lunch decline in memory scores by 58 percent compared with the high-carb meals. Both lunch groups had similar declines in attention.

British Journal of Nutrition, February 2017

Chocolate Slows Cognitive Decline for Some

The good news for chocolate lovers just keeps coming. A new longitudinal prospective study looked at the relationship between chocolate consumption and cognitive decline in an elderly cognitively healthy population. The 531 participants, ages 65 and over, initially had normal Mini-Mental State Examination (MMSE) scores, and their dietary habits were evaluated at the study's start. After an average follow-up of 48 months, the MMSE test was given again, with cognitive decline defined as a decrease of two or more points from the initial score. Results were adjusted for age, education, smoking, alcohol drinking, body mass index, hypertension, and diabetes. Chocolate intake was associated with a 41 percent lower risk of cognitive decline. But this protective effect was observed only among subjects with an average daily consumption of caffeine lower than 75 milligrams (69 percent of the participants)—less than found in a single typical cup of coffee. The researchers concluded, "To our knowledge, this is the first prospective cohort study to show an inverse association between regular long-term chocolate consumption and cognitive decline in humans."

Journal of Alzheimer's Disease, May 6, 2016

Benefits of Chocolate

The ancient Olmec, Mayan, and Aztec peoples were onto something about the benefits of chocolate when they began consuming it, mostly in the form of cocoa beverages, some 3,500 years ago. Today science is finding that phytochemical compounds called flavanols found in dark chocolate (the darker, the better) and cocoa have cardiovascular benefits. But in news that cheered chocoholics everywhere, those same compounds also may be good for your brain. Most recently, scientists published the first prospective cohort study to show an inverse association between regular long-term chocolate consumption and cognitive decline in humans (see Box 4-4, "Chocolate Slows Cognitive Decline for Some").

Also making headlines and garnering cheers from chocolate lovers was the 2016 Maine-Syracuse Longitudinal Study. Involving 968 participants ranging from 23 to 98 years old, the study linked frequent chocolate consumption to benefits for neurocognition and behavior. Habitual chocolate intake was related to cognitive performance, measured with an extensive battery of neuropsychological tests. More frequent chocolate consumption was significantly associated with better performance on overall composite scores and the Mini-Mental State Examination. Chocolate eaters also did better on specific tests of visual-spatial memory and organization, working memory, scanning and tracking, and abstract reasoning.

Making Your Brain Work Better

Dark chocolate might also have benefits for specific mental functions, even in the short term, according to a study published in 2015. The eight-week study of 90 cognitively healthy older volunteers randomly assigned to three different levels of cocoa flavanols found improvements in verbal fluency and tests of visual attention and task switching, with greater benefits associated with higher amounts. Both the high- and intermediate-flavanol beverages were associated with significantly greater improvements in scores, compared to the low-flavanol drink.

In another study, a chocolate drink high in flavanols enabled participants to complete memory-related tasks with less effort. The randomized trial compared three strengths of flavanol-laden beverages on 63 volunteers, ages 40 to 65, over a 30-day period. No difference was seen in tests of mental accuracy and reaction time. But, while performing the memory-related tasks, during which their brain activity was monitored with CT scans, participants in the middle and top groups of flavanol supplementation required less brain activity to accomplish the tasks than those in the lowest group. According to a study of people in Luxemburg, chocolate also may improve insulin resistance, which could in turn help protect the heart and brain.

Cocoa Effective Against Impairment

Other findings suggest that cocoa may have greater benefits for people who have already suffered cognitive impairments than those who are cognitively healthy, although others report preventive benefits. In one Italian clinical trial, for example, older adults with mild cognitive impairment improved their scores on some mental tests when they consumed cocoa flavanols. Importantly, researchers noted, the improvements in cognitive function were seen over a relatively short period of time, just eight weeks.

Another study tested the effects of cocoa consumption in 60 volunteers, average age 73, who had hypertension and/or diabetes. Although none had dementia, 17 suffered from a condition called impaired neurovascular coupling (NVC), a measure of blood flow in the brain as it relates to nerve cells (neurons). Researchers initially tested two levels of flavanols in cocoa, consumed twice a day for 30 days. Participants were encouraged to alter their diets to compensate for the extra calories in the cocoa. No significant differences were seen between the two types of cocoa, so the results from both groups were merged. Participants free of impaired NVC showed no significant benefits from cocoa consumption. But the small group of volunteers with impaired NVC saw dramatic changes after just a month of cocoa intake: Neurovascular coupling improved by more than double, and scores on standard cognitive tests jumped 30 percent.

Chocolate Choices

Cocoa flavanols also are associated with improvements in blood pressure, blood glucose, and insulin resistance. So it isn't clear whether the benefits in cognition seen in such studies are a direct consequence of cocoa flavanols or a secondary effect of these general improvements in health.

If you do decide to up your chocolate intake in hopes of brain benefits, keep in mind that chocolate has plenty of calories and often comes with lots of added sugar and saturated fats. Finding chocolate choices high in flavanols can be a challenge, adds Jeffrey Blumberg, PhD, director of Tufts' HNRCA Antioxidants Research Laboratory: "The FDA does not require food producers to list the content of flavonoids, such as those that give dark chocolate its health benefits, in the Nutrition Facts panel or elsewhere on the label. Moreover, because of lawsuits, some products that used to cite their 'flavonoid' or 'flavanol' or 'natural antioxidant' content (e.g., on chocolate and tea) no longer do so. Because there is no reference standard (RDA or DV) for flavonoids, per FDA guidelines no product can claim to be a good or rich source of them."

Benefits of Coffee

Another product once thought to be an indulgence to limit or avoid that's now been shown to have health benefits is coffee. The 2015 Dietary Guidelines Advisory Committee concluded that coffee is safe to drink at typical levels of consumption, and suggested it could actually have health benefits. For example, a large Korean study reported that people drinking three to five cups of coffee daily were 41 percent less likely to show signs of coronary artery calcium than non-coffee drinkers. This calcification is an early indicator of the artery-clogging plaques that characterize atherosclerosis. The study, published in *Heart*, may help explain one mechanism by which coffee benefits the cardiovascular system. Previous studies, the researchers noted, have linked coffee consumption to improved insulin sensitivity and reduced oxidation of LDL cholesterol (oxidation makes these particles more dangerous). Findings on coffee and coronary artery calcium, however, have

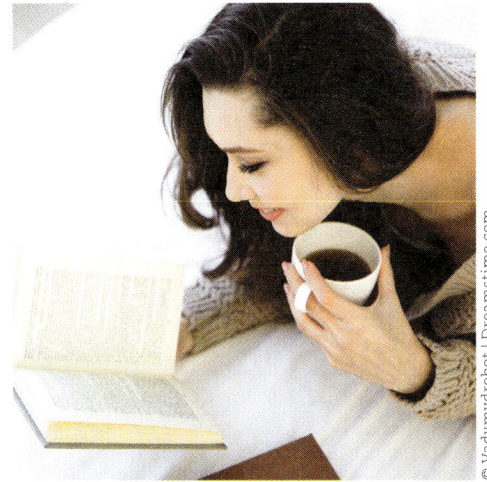

BOX 4-5

For Older Women, More Caffeine May Mean Less Dementia Risk

Part of the apparent cognitive protection associated with drinking coffee may be due to the caffeine content, according to a new study of 6,467 older women. Self-reported caffeine consumption of more than 261 milligrams of caffeine (about that in three cups of coffee or five to six cups of black tea) was associated with a 36 percent lower risk of dementia over 10 years of follow-up. The study was unusual because it afforded an opportunity to analyze over time the relationships between caffeine intake and dementia incidence in a large group of women who consumed different levels of caffeine. Consumption was estimated from questions about coffee, tea, and cola beverage intake, including frequency and serving size. Participants were part of the Women's Health Initiative Memory Study funded by the National Heart, Lung, and Blood Institute; over 10 years, 388 of the women were diagnosed with probable dementia or some form of global cognitive impairment. Researchers cautioned that the observational study can't prove cause and effect. But they pointed out that caffeine binds to adenosine receptors in the brain, so the findings point to a potential mechanism worth further investigating, adding, "The mounting evidence of caffeine consumption as a potentially protective factor against cognitive impairment is exciting given that caffeine is also an easily modifiable dietary factor."

The Journals of Gerontology, Series A: Biological Sciences and Medical Sciences, Sept. 27, 2016

been mixed, possibly because prior studies had a lag time of seven to eight years between measures of coffee intake and subsequent calcification.

Some studies as well as popular lore, however, had raised the possibility that coffee might raise the risk of atrial fibrillation ("afib")—heart "flutters" that can be serious. But a Chinese study put that notion to the test by combining the findings from a half-dozen prior observational studies totaling nearly 230,000 participants. Publishing their analysis in the *Canadian Journal of Cardiology,* the researchers reported that participants grouped as high caffeine consumers—more than 500 milligrams daily, or about six cups of American coffee—were actually less likely (16 percent) to develop afib. With each additional regular daily intake of 300 milligrams of caffeine, afib risk declined 6 percent.

Coffee contains a wealth of phytochemicals with possible cardiovascular benefits. In turn, these are probably also important to brain health.

Caffeine Effects

Coffee is also a leading source of caffeine, and other benefits from coffee consumption, perhaps not surprisingly, are associated with its caffeine content. Researchers have tested mice given water spiked with caffeine—the human equivalent of about five cups of coffee a day—versus mice given plain water to drink. The mice had been specially bred to develop an Alzheimer's-like disease. After several months, the mice that received only water had difficulty navigating in mazes, while the caffeinated mice easily found their way out of the mazes.

Studies in humans have found that caffeine consumption in midlife may help to protect against cognitive decline later in life. Recent results from the Baltimore Longitudinal Study of Aging showed that caffeine intake was associated with better baseline global cognition among participants age 70 and older.

Another study concluded that older women who drank at least three cups of coffee daily were 18 percent less likely to develop problems with verbal recall and 33 percent less prone to memory problems than those who drank less coffee. Similar results were seen for tea, leading researchers to identify caffeine as the source of the benefit. Other evidence suggests caffeine intake may be tied to a lower risk of dementia (see box 4-5 "For Older Women, More Caffeine May Mean Less Dementia Risk").

Coffee could also help ward off depression. A Harvard study reported that women consuming two or three cups of regular coffee per day were 15% less likely to develop depression over a follow-up period of 10 years than those drinking one cup a day or less. Those drinking four cups a day were at 20% lower risk.

Don't Add Calories to Your Coffee

If you're drinking coffee in part for its brain benefits, make sure you're not canceling out those positives by dosing your cup with extra calories. You may not give much thought to adding a splash of cream and a spoonful of sugar to your coffee or tea, but these add-ins can add up in calories. A study published in *Public Health* aimed to figure out just how much.

Scientists analyzed data gathered in the National Health and Nutrition Examination Survey (NHANES) from 13,185 coffee drinkers and 6,215 tea consumers over about a decade.

Based on self-reports of what people drank over a 24-hour period, it was calculated that drinking coffee with caloric add-ins was, on average, associated with a daily increase of 69 calories compared to drinking it black. Drinking tea with add-ins resulted in an average daily increase of 43 calories compared to plain tea. With both beverages, sugar contributed the most to calories from add-ins and amounted to an average of 2 to 2½ teaspoons daily. Dairy add-ins increased saturated fat intake.

"Consider gradually reducing, then eventually omitting, sugar and sugary syrups in these drinks, and replace cream with low-fat or skim milk," says Ruopeng An, PhD, the lead author of the study at the University of Illinois at Urbana-Champaign.

Benefits of Tea

Similarly, tea might benefit the brain in many different ways. Jeffrey Blumberg, PhD, senior scientist at Tufts' HNRCA Antioxidants Research Laboratory, says, "As investigators continue to study the multiple effects that tea has on human health, more research supports tea's potential in helping reduce the incidence of major diseases. In some respect, it is good to think of tea as a plant food."

Studies support cognitive benefits from most types of tea, but especially green tea. All tea comes from the leaves of the *Camellia sinensis* bush. Green tea is unfermented and minimally processed, the leaves simply withered and steamed. Black tea is fermented and oxidized. Oolong tea is partly oxidized, between green and black tea. White tea is made from partly opened buds and young leaves, which are steamed and dried. (Herbal "tea" is not actually made from tea leaves, but may have health benefits nonetheless—see below.)

One small clinical trial reported that green tea improves the connectivity between parts of the brain involved in tasks of "working memory." Swiss researchers tested the effects of a beverage containing 27.5 grams of green-tea extract (equivalent to about two cups of brewed green tea) against a placebo. Healthy young male volunteers were then faced with a battery of working-memory tasks, while their brains were monitored using magnetic resonance imaging. Men who had been given the beverage containing green-tea extract showed increased connectivity between the brain's right superior parietal lobe and the frontal cortex. This effect on connectivity within the brain coincided with improvements in actual cognitive performance on working-memory exercises.

In another study of people with mild memory impairment, daily supplements of green tea extract plus L-theanine (an amino acid unique to tea) over four months improved memory and mental alertness compared to a placebo.

Polyphenols in Tea

Like other plants, tea is a rich source of phytochemicals, including compounds called phytochemicals. One reason green tea might be especially

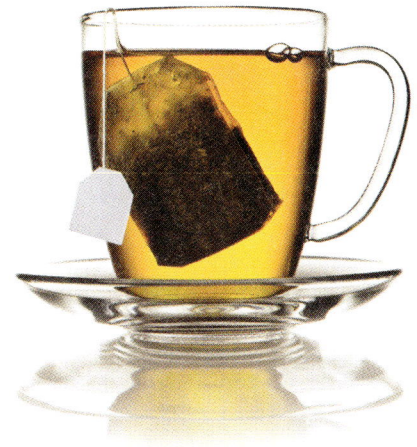

good for your brain is that it contains a polyphenol compound called EGCG (epigallocatechin-3-gallate). Researchers at the University of Michigan have reported that EGCG prevents the formation of potentially dangerous amyloid aggregates associated with the development of Alzheimer's disease. A green-tea extract also broke down existing aggregates in proteins that contained metals—copper, iron, and zinc—associated with the disease.

British scientists have tested the effect of green tea extracts on "balls" of amyloid proteins created in the lab. The extracts caused the shape of the balls to distort in such a way that they could no longer bind to nerve cells and disrupt their functioning.

Tea and Blood Pressure

Another way drinking tea might benefit your brain is by keeping a lid on high blood pressure, which is the number-one risk factor for strokes and vascular dementia. One Australian study reported that drinking three cups daily of regular black tea was associated with a small but significant drop in blood pressure. Researchers divided 95 study participants, ages 35 to 75, into two groups: One group drank three cups of black tea daily, while a control group drank a placebo beverage containing the same amount of caffeine but no actual tea. At the study's start, participants had systolic blood pressure readings ranging from 115 to 150 mmHg (normal to stage-one hypertension). After six months, those in the tea-drinking group saw an average drop in systolic pressure (the top number) of two to three points and about a two-point drop in diastolic pressure, compared to the control group.

Although those improvements are small, researchers said they had important potential public-health benefits: "At a population level, the observed differences in blood pressure would be associated with a 10 percent reduction in the prevalence of hypertension and a 7 percent to 10 percent reduction in the risk of heart disease and stroke."

Hibiscus vs. Hypertension

Herbal teas may have their own blood-pressure benefits. Hibiscus is one of the most common ingredients in herbal teas; it gives the beverages a fruity, tart taste and red color. This fruit of a flowering plant is rich in antioxidants including anthocyanins, flavones, flavonols, and phenolic acids. Research led by Diane L. McKay, PhD, of Tufts' HNRCA Antioxidants Research Laboratory, has shown that a few cups a day of herbal-tea-containing hibiscus can help to lower high blood pressure in pre-hypertensive and mildly hypertensive adults as effectively as some medications do.

In one study, Dr. McKay and colleagues recruited 65 pre- or mildly hypertensive volunteers, ages 30 to 70. About half of the participants drank three cups of hibiscus tea per day for six weeks, while a control group received a placebo beverage containing artificial hibiscus flavoring and color. Those who drank the hibiscus tea saw a 7.2-point drop in their systolic blood pressure, significantly more than the placebo group. Those results are comparable to that delivered by standard blood-pressure medications. Participants with the highest blood pressure at the study's start showed the most significant reductions.

Wine and Resveratrol Research

Another "plant food" consumed as a beverage that is being studied for brain benefits is wine (along with grape juice). One focus of such research is a compound called resveratrol, found in red wine and grape juice, a type of polyphenol produced as part of a plant's defense system against disease. Resveratrol is also found in dark chocolate.

German researchers tested supplements of 200 milligrams of resveratrol daily for six months versus a placebo in 46 cognitively healthy people, ages 50 to 80. At the end of the study, participants randomly assigned to the resveratrol supplements scored better on memory tests and showed greater functional connectivity in their brains.

Action Against Alzheimer's

Scientists have shown that the polyphenols in red wine block the formation of proteins that contribute to the development of the toxic plaques found in the brains of individuals with Alzheimer's disease. These red-wine compounds also reduce the toxicity of existing plaques. Natural chemicals found in red wine as well as in green tea can interrupt the process by which Alzheimer's proteins latch onto brain cells.

Keep in mind, however, that research on resveratrol is in the very early stages, and it may be that benefits are associated only with amounts impossible to consume except from supplements. That is the case, for example, of recent research on resveratrol and changes in the brain associated with Alzheimer's disease. Resveratrol stabilized the levels of beta-amyloid protein in patients given two grams daily—the equivalent of the amount in 1,000 bottles of wine. The year-long study recruited 119 people with diagnoses of probable Alzheimer's. As the disease progresses, beta-amyloid levels ordinarily drop as the proteins are converted into toxic plaques in the brain. But in patients randomly assigned to resveratrol, that decline slowed—possibly, scientists suggested, because resveratrol stimulates enzymes that slow metabolism and cellular aging. Researchers cautioned that further investigation is needed to determine whether resveratrol has a beneficial effect, and that the results don't mean people should begin taking supplements.

Like all alcoholic beverages, moreover, wine should be consumed only in moderation—no more than two glasses a day for men and one for women.

Don't Forget Water

While drinking cocoa, coffee, tea, and wine may have brain benefits, the most important beverage for your brain is plain old water—and you might not be getting enough. Older people may be less sensitive to thirst, so it's especially important for them to stay hydrated.

Dehydration has negative effects on your mood and cognitive performance, including memory, attention, and motor skills. Research on hydration and brain function—especially on positive effects of drinking more fluids—is limited and contradictory, however. The safest bet is to make sure you drink plenty of fluids (coffee and tea count, too) that don't add calories, and to pay attention to your body's thirst signals.

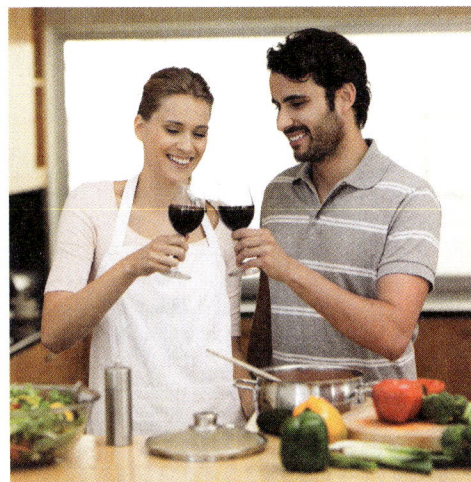

Should You Avoid Diet Soda?

A startling 10-year study of participants in the Framingham Heart Study reported that those who drank diet soda daily were almost three times as likely to suffer a stroke and develop dementia as those who consumed it weekly or less. The study followed 2,888 participants, ages 45 and older, for stroke incidence and 1,484 Framingham participants, ages 60 and up, for dementia. They consumed artificial sweeteners including saccharin, acesulfame-K, and aspartame; more recently approved sweeteners, such as sucralose, neotame, and stevia, were not represented. Researchers emphasized that the study showed only correlation, not causation, but suggested people should be "cautious" about their diet soda intake; it's possible, for instance, that people already at greater risk because of diabetes or obesity were more likely to consume diet drinks. Scientists added that the results should not cause people to switch to sugary sodas, which were not linked to greater risk. (That could be because participants did not drink sugary beverages as often.) Other experts pointed out the absence of a dose-response effect: In fact, while those who drank one diet soda a day were three times more likely to develop dementia, those drinking two to six per day did not have an increased risk over those drinking zero artificially sweetened drinks.

Stroke, May 2017

Fish Benefits Outweigh Mercury Concerns

Scientists who examined autopsied brain tissue from 286 people who had reported their seafood intake an average of 4.5 years before their deaths may have new clues about the benefits and risks of consuming seafood. Researchers found that older adults who ate more seafood, which can contain mercury, had higher brain levels of mercury—but that toxin was not associated with any signs of dementia. On the other hand, people at greatest genetic risk for Alzheimer's who consumed the most seafood showed less evidence of the disease's damage in the brain. The participants in Rush University's Memory and Aging Project were initially free of dementia; average age at death was almost 90. The protective benefits of seafood consumption were limited to participants with the ApoE4 genetic variant linked to increased risk of developing Alzheimer's disease. But scientists speculated that this increased risk made it easier to detect a strong difference between the brains of those who did and did not frequently eat seafood. People without the genetic variant might have had too little Alzheimer's proteins in their brains to detect.

JAMA, February 2, 2016

Another reason to prefer water for hydration is that some concerns have been raised about negative effects of the sweeteners used in diet sodas. While it's too soon to say you should swear off these beverages, water is always a smart choice (see Box 4-6, "Should You Avoid Diet Soda?").

Seafood and Cognition

Seafood, especially the fatty varieties high in fish oil (heart-healthy omega-3s), seems to have brain benefits. Even if you've never been a big seafood eater, it's not too late to reduce your risk of cognitive impairment and dementia by eating more fish. In fact, a recent study reports that this dietary change may be more beneficial later in life. Chinese researchers reported that age significantly modify the association between fish consumption and cognitive change: Among adults ages 65 and older, those who ate one or more weekly serving of fish saw a slower rate of cognitive decline compared to those consuming less fish. The difference was equivalent to what would be expected from 1.6 years of difference in age. Fish consumption was also associated with a slower decline in composite and verbal memory scores. No associations were observed, however, among those ages 55 to 64.

People at higher risk of developing Alzheimer's because of genetic factors might also benefit more from eating more fish. Carriers of the APOE4 genetic factor for Alzheimer's disease might be able to reduce their risk simply by eating more fish, according to data from the Rush Memory and Aging Project. Higher seafood intake was also associated with greater brain levels of mercury, found in some fish varieties, but this was not linked to neuropathology. An accompanying editorial noted that the results suggest that seafood "can be consumed without substantial concern of mercury contamination diminishing its possible cognitive benefit in older adults" (see Box 4-7, "Fish Benefits Outweigh Mercury Concerns").

The Role of Omega-3s

Fatty acids play an important role in brain health, so it makes sense that seafood rich in the omega-3 fatty acids eicosapentaenoic acid (EPA) and docosahexaenioc acid (DHA) could be good for your brain. DHA is the most prominent fatty acid in the brain, especially in the neurons of the cerebral cortex—the brain's grey matter responsible for memory, language, and thinking.

The importance of omega-3s in general and DHA in particular to seafood's cognitive effects was demonstrated in a Tufts study several years ago. It involved nearly 900 elderly men and women initially free of dementia, who were screened for cognitive decline every two years. Following up an average nine years later, the researchers documented 99 cases of dementia, including 71 with Alzheimer's disease.

Among the 488 participants who also completed a dietary questionnaire, those with the highest blood DHA levels reported that they ate

BOX 4-8

an average of nearly three fish servings a week. Participants with lower DHA levels ate substantially less fish. Those with higher blood levels of DHA, as well as those eating the most fish, had a dramatically lower risk of dementia and Alzheimer's disease. Subjects with the highest DHA levels had a 47 percent reduced risk of dementia and a 39 percent lower risk of Alzheimer's.

Though a form of omega-3 called alpha-linolenic acid (ALA) found in plants can be converted in your body to the more complex types found in fish, this conversion is not very efficient. The best way to obtain EPA and DHA is to consume fish, especially fatty varieties such as salmon, sardines, and mackerel (see Box 4-8, "Shopping for Seafood").

Are fish-oil pills, which also contain EPA and DHA, as beneficial as eating fish? We'll weigh the evidence in the next chapter. But nothing beats eating more fish—in part because of what you *don't* eat when fish is the entrée: Dining on salmon instead of a ribeye steak gives you healthy fat instead of saturated fat.

Gray Matter and Fish

People who eat more fish also literally have more grey matter than non-fish eaters. In a study using MRI scans, people eating broiled or baked fish, but not fried fish, on a weekly basis had greater volumes of gray matter in the brain's hippocampus and frontal and temporal lobes. In subsequent cognitive testing, only 3.2 percent of those with the highest fish intake and greatest preservation of gray matter developed mild cognitive impairment or dementia. That was a sharp contrast to the 30.8 percent of non-fish eaters who'd suffered such cognitive decline. Average scores for working memory were significantly better among weekly fish eaters, too.

Researchers concluded, "Consuming baked or broiled fish promotes stronger neurons in the brain's grey matter by making them larger and healthier. This simple lifestyle choice increases the brain's resistance to Alzheimer's disease and lowers risk for the disorder."

Fish Smarts

That's not the only study to find that baked and broiled (or grilled) fish are more beneficial than fried fish. This is likely due to the extra calories and saturated or *trans* fat added to fried fish in the breading and frying process. The type of fish commonly used for frying may also be a factor: Cod and other whitefish varieties are much lower in omega-3 content than other types of fish.

Shellfish generally falls short on omega-3s, too. Although shrimp, for example, is a lean source of high-quality protein, it is low in total fat and thus also low in omega-3 fatty acids. The omega-3 content of crab is somewhat higher, similar to that of canned light tuna, although it varies widely by species.

The recommendations to eat more seafood remain a work in progress, much like other links between specific types of food and cognition. No single food or group of foods is a "magic bullet" against Alzheimer's and dementia, but the right food choices, as part of an overall healthy dietary pattern, can nonetheless help improve your odds.

Shopping for Seafood

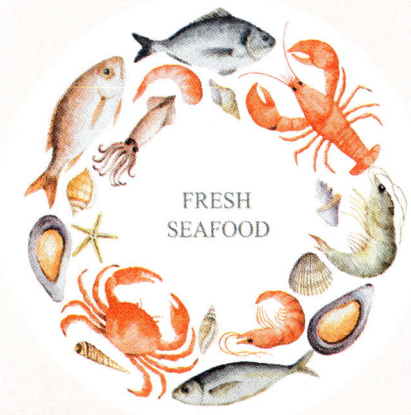

FRESH SEAFOOD

© Elena Medvedeva | Dreamstime.com

Fish highest in omega-3 fatty acids that also are rated high for sustainability (notes in parentheses) include:

- Arctic char (farmed)
- Bluefish
- Herring (Atlantic)
- Mackerel ((U.S., Canada wild-caught)
- Opah (Hawaii)
- Sablefish
- Salmon (other than farmed Atlantic)
- Sardines (Pacific)
- Striped bass
- Swordfish (not imported)
- Trout (not Lake Huron or Lake Michigan)
- Tuna (Albacore)

Nearly all fish and shellfish contain traces of mercury. For most people, according to the FDA, the risk from mercury by eating fish and shellfish is not a health concern; the exceptions are women who might become pregnant, women who are pregnant, nursing mothers, and young children.

NUTRITION FOR YOUR BRAIN FROM PILLS

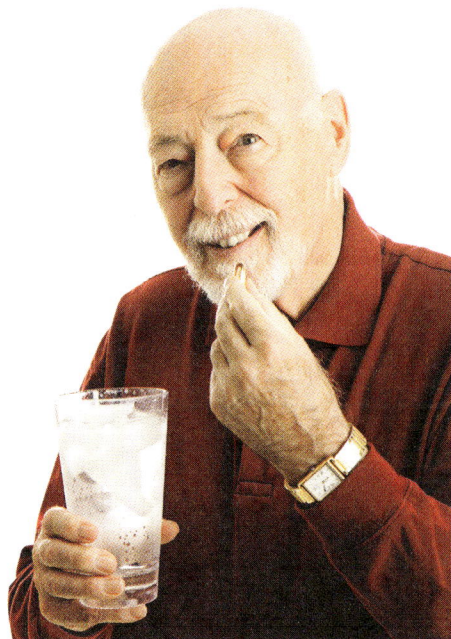

© Lisa F. Young | Dreamstime.com

Insurance from Multivitamins

Americans have been taking multivitamin/mineral supplements since the early 1940s, and an estimated one-third of all U.S. consumers take them regularly as insurance against nutritional shortfalls. Multivitamins account for almost one-sixth of all purchases of dietary supplements and 40 percent of all sales of vitamin and mineral supplements—nearly $6 billion annually.

Taking a pill containing the nutrients believed to be beneficial for your brain, such as those found in a multivitamin or in various specific supplements, should logically have the same effects as eating healthy foods. Many studies testing that premise for other health benefits, however, have proven disappointing. For reasons scientists can't fully explain, vitamins and minerals consumed in whole foods seem to affect the body differently than when popped in pill form. It may be that synergistic relationships between nutrients trigger benefits that are not present in isolation.

Research on Multivitamins

One of the largest clinical trials to look at whether the combination of vitamins and minerals in a daily multivitamin might help protect your aging brain used data from the Physicians' Health Study II. Participants were 5,947 men, average age 71.6, who were randomly assigned to receive either a daily multivitamin or a placebo. The analysis combined five tests of global cognitive function as well as testing verbal memory. Over an average follow-up of 8.5 years, changes in mental function were no different in the multivitamin group than in those taking a placebo. Researchers concluded, "These data do not provide support for use of multivitamin supplements in the prevention of cognitive decline."

Benefits of Fish Oil

One of the key benefit of eating fish is increasing your intake of DHA and EPA, the two most important omega-3s found in fish. This leads to the question of whether taking a fish-oil pill would have similar brain benefits? This question has been more extensively studied than most promises of brain benefits from supplements, but to date, the evidence is mixed, at best.

Recently, one of the largest and longest studies of its kind, a five-year clinical trial with more than 3,000 participants, reported no benefits from omega-3 supplements against cognitive decline. In addition to disappointing findings for fish-oil pills, the study also found no benefits compared to placebo from supplements of lutein and zeaxanthin, two carotenoid compounds found in green, leafy vegetables. Researchers took advantage of data from the Age-Related Eye Disease Study 2 (AREDS2), which was a follow-up to groundbreaking research from AREDS1 that showed a combination of antioxidant vitamins could help prevent age-related macular degeneration (AMD). AREDS2 tested the addition of DHA/EPA (1 milligram daily) as well as lutein (10 milligrams) and zeaxanthin (2 milligrams). Because many of the participants agreed to a battery of cognitive tests every two years, the data from the vision research also could be used to look for brain benefits.

Because of the makeup of the study population, however, this otherwise-definitive-seeming research may not yet be the final word. Participants post came from a well-nourished, highly educated population, and it could be that supplementing the already healthy diet of highly educated individuals isn't going to have much added benefit on cognition.

Scanning for Benefits

Another study that used brain scans did report a benefit from fish-oil pills. Researchers took a retrospective look at the effects of fish-oil supplements on brain activity and behavior in 819 older adults who participated in the Alzheimer's Disease Neuroimaging Initiative. Every six months, participants completed standard cognitive tests for memory and other mental abilities and underwent brain magnetic resonance imaging (MRI) scans. Individuals who took fish-oil pills had significantly less brain atrophy and better scores on cognitive tests than those not taking the supplements. But these beneficial effects were seen only in those with normal cognitive abilities when the study started. Participants who already displayed mild cognitive impairments or Alzheimer's saw no improvement from taking the supplements.

Omega-3s in the Brain

Why might extra omega-3s benefit the brain? Lipids, a collective term for fats and oils, make up about 50 to 60 percent of the brain's dry weight, and the omega-3 fatty acid DHA, which is found in fish oil, is the most abundant fatty acid found in the nerve cell membrane. However, as a result of the cumulative effects of oxidative damage, the DHA composition of the brain decreases with age.

It may be that taking extra DHA in pill form can slow this decrease and protect cognitive functioning. Among healthy older adults not already suffering cognitive decline, randomized controlled trials have shown that supplements of DHA (800 to 900 milligrams/day) can improve verbal, visuospatial, and episodic memory. A lower dose of DHA—similar to that in most commercial fish-oil supplements—did not influence cognitive function, however.

On the other hand, a review of three high-quality clinical trials totaling 3,536 participants found no significant differences in the performance of cognitive tasks between individuals taking fish-oil supplements or placebo. Again, doses were relatively low—ranging from 400 to 700 milligrams daily. Only small, insignificant improvements in performance on tests of memory, executive function, and mental processing speed were found for individuals given fish-oil supplements.

Fish-Oil Pills May Improve Mild Cognitive Impairment

Although results for omega-3 fish-oil supplements on brainpower are mixed, a new Chinese study offers some reason for optimism. Scientists investigated the effects of omega-3 supplements on 86 older Chinese men and women, average age 71, who were already suffering from mild cognitive impairment (MCI). Roughly half the participants were randomly assigned to receive daily supplements of 480 milligrams of DHA and 720 milligrams of EPA, the two primary omega-3s in fish oil; the rest were assigned to receive an olive oil placebo. After six months, supplementation was associated with improved scores on Basic Cognitive Aptitude Tests (BCAT), better perceptual speed, space imagery efficiency, and working memory. Two other cognitive measures, mental arithmetic efficiency and recognition memory, were not improved in the intervention group. The researchers also noted several gender differences in the effects of the omega-3 supplements. They concluded, "Omega-3 fatty acids can improve cognitive function in people with MCI. Further studies with different fish oil dosages, longer intervention periods, and larger sample sizes should be investigated before definite recommendations can be made."

Nutrients, January 2017

B Vitamin Effects Don't Translate to Brain

While vitamin B supplements can reduce levels of homocysteine, an amino acid associated with greater risk of cognitive impairment, hopes that the pills might also have brain benefits keep getting dashed. A new meta-analysis pooled four clinical trials testing supplements of folic acid along with vitamin B12 and/or vitamin B6. The intervention groups receiving extra B vitamins saw significantly lowered homocysteine levels than the control groups, which might be expected to be associated with accompanying cognitive effects. But testing using the standard Mini-Mental State Examination (MMSE) failed to find any significant difference between the groups, despite the supplements and reduced homocysteine levels.

Journal of Geriatric Psychology and Neurology, January 2017

Effects Against Impairment

The evidence is even still more limited for the benefits of fish-oil supplements among people already diagnosed with mild cognitive impairment or Alzheimer's. Only a few small studies have suggested that omega-3 supplements help these patients any more than a placebo. One Chinese study recently reported improvements from omega-3 supplementation in people already suffering mild cognitive impairment (see Box 5-1, "Fish-Oil Pills May Improve Mild Cognitive Impairment"). Another small pilot study found that large doses of DHA, along with EPA and other compounds touted for brain benefits, improved cognition as well as frailty among older women. Because of the mixture of supplements, however, it's impossible to say whether the benefits were due to the omega-3s or to other ingredients.

A small study in Japan looked at the effects of omega-3 DHA plus ARA (arachidonic acid), an omega-6 fatty acid, in patients with mild cognitive impairment. After 90 days, those who received supplements rather than a placebo showed significant improvements in immediate memory and attention. Those whose cognitive impairment was due to brain lesions improved the most, but those with early Alzheimer's disease did not benefit from the supplements.

If you don't enjoy eating seafood or you are a vegan or vegetarian, it may be tempting to pop a pill instead of consuming salmon and other fatty fish. But don't count on the pills to protect your brain—the evidence is still mixed and research is ongoing.

Vitamin B12 Deficiency

As with omega-3s, it makes biological sense that taking supplemental B vitamins would benefit your brain, and indeed some of the earliest research on vitamin B12 deficiency connected it to central-nervous-system problems. Vitamins B6 and B12 and folate are critical components of a metabolic cycle important for DNA synthesis. Deficiencies of these vitamins are associated with high levels of homocysteine, an amino acid associated with cardiovascular disease that may also be linked to cerebrovascular disease, including stroke and vascular dementia. Some studies have also found high levels of homocysteine in the brains of Alzheimer's patients.

But taking B vitamin supplements, even when they succeed in lowering homocysteine levels, doesn't necessarily protect the brain. The evidence from such studies is complex and even contradictory (see Box 5-2,"B Vitamin Effects Don't Translate to Brain").

For example, Dutch researchers studied 2,919 people, average age 74, with elevated levels of homocysteine. Participants were randomly assigned to a placebo or a daily tablet containing 400 micrograms of folic acid and 500 micrograms of vitamin B12. Participants given the supplements saw their homocysteine levels decline almost four times as much as that of the control group. But after two years, cognitive scores between the two groups on a battery of tests differed only slightly.

B12 Deficiency and Cognition

Research does show that cognitive decline is likely associated with vitamin B12 deficiency. One study found that people with insufficient levels of B12 were at greater risk of cognitive decline over nearly five years of follow-up than those with adequate levels of the vitamin. Very low levels of B12 also predicted decreased total brain volume. Another study reported that older people with low—but still normal—blood levels of B12 were six times more likely to experience brain atrophy compared to those with the highest blood levels of the vitamin.

This could be of particular concern for older adults, who often have difficulty absorbing B12 from food because of changes to the gastrointestinal system due to aging. Certain medications, such as stomach-acid blockers, can also contribute to the risk of B12 deficiency. Federal dietary guidelines recommend that people age 50 and older consume foods fortified with vitamin B12 and/or B12 supplements (see Box 5-3, "Foods High in Vitamin B12").

Even a Little Low Raises Risk

Tufts scientists have found that even if you're only a little low in vitamin B12, you might be at greater risk for cognitive decline than previously thought. Their study divided 549 participants, average age 75, into five groups based on their blood levels of vitamin B12. Men and women in the second-lowest group did not fare any better in terms of cognitive decline than those at the bottom of vitamin B12 blood levels. Over an eight-year period, scores on Mini-Mental State Examination (MMSE) tests declined slightly overall. But average declines were significantly faster in both the lowest and second-lowest groups ranked by vitamin B12 status.

"While we emphasize our study does not show causation, the associations which were found raise the concern that some of the cognitive decline seen in older adults may be the result of inadequate vitamin B12 in older adults for whom maintaining normal blood levels can be a challenge," says senior author Paul F. Jacques, DSc.

Pills Unproven

Since vitamin B12 deficiency is associated with poorer cognition, it makes sense that B vitamin supplements might help protect the brain. But giving people extra B vitamin supplements has not always paid dividends in brain health.

A recent English double-blind, randomized trial tested vitamin B12 supplements against a placebo in 201 patients with an average age of 75, who had a moderate B12 deficiency. After one year, vitamin B12 status in the intervention group improved dramatically. But there was no evidence of an effect on cognitive function or nerve or motor functions. Researchers concluded: "Results of the trial do not support the hypothesis that the correction of moderate vitamin B12 deficiency, in the absence of anemia and of neurologic and cognitive signs or

BOX 5-3

Foods High in Vitamin B12

© Nina Pyankova | Dreamstime.com

These food servings all provide at least 25 percent of the Daily Value of vitamin B12:

- Clams, cooked, 3 oz.
- Rainbow trout, 3 oz.
- Sockeye salmon, 3 oz.
- Lean top sirloin, broiled, 3 oz.
- Plain skim yogurt, 1 cup
- Fortified breakfast cereal, 1 cup

symptoms, has beneficial effects on neurologic or cognitive function in later life."

Subgroup Effects

So it could be that extra B vitamins benefit only certain subgroups of people, such as those initially with a low intake of B vitamins or elevated homocysteine levels. One positive study, dubbed VITACOG, compared the effects of high-dose B-complex supplements and placebo in older adults. Those given the extra B vitamins experienced slower brain atrophy. As in other studies, the benefits were greatest among subjects with elevated blood levels of homocysteine.

A British study also reported that supplemental doses of folate, B6, and B12 were associated with significantly less brain atrophy over time compared to placebo. Greater rates of brain atrophy were associated with lower cognitive test scores at the end of the study.

Recent research has also suggested that genetic factors may influence the interaction between cognitive performance and B vitamin status.

Best Advice for Now

Until we know more, make sure that you're consuming adequate amounts of B vitamins from foods (consider adding fortified foods and supplements to your diet, if necessary, if you're over age 50). But don't bother taking mega-doses in hopes of turning back the clock on your brain.

In fact, too much of a good thing—folate, another important B vitamin—might actually be bad for your brain, according to an Australian study. Participants with low vitamin B12 and high folate levels were more than three times as likely to have impaired cognitive performance as those with normal levels. Participants with high folate levels, but normal vitamin B12, were also somewhat more likely to have impaired cognitive performance.

Vitamin D, Beyond the Hype

Although recent studies on many of the hoped-for benefits of extra vitamin D have been disappointing, it's nonetheless important for your brain to make sure you're getting enough of the "sunshine vitamin." Researchers at Rutgers and the University of California-Davis compared blood levels of vitamin D in 318 adults, average age 76, with changes in cognition over five years. Those with low vitamin D levels were more likely to decline faster on tests of memory and executive function than those with normal levels. That rate of decline, related to vitamin D status, was similar for those with normal cognition at the start of the study and those already suffering some impairment. At the start of the study, moreover, participants who already had dementia were more likely to have low vitamin D levels. Initial vitamin D deficiency was also associated with poorer semantic memory (remembering general information), visuospatial ability, and executive function.

It can be challenging to determine whether low levels of vitamin D are the cause of health problems or an effect of poor health and aging. Older

Participants who already had dementia were more likely to have low vitamin D levels.

adults and people in poor health often have trouble consuming adequate nutrients and spend less time outdoors in the sun. The skin naturally synthesizes vitamin D when exposed to sunlight—hence the "sunshine vitamin" nickname. If you're stuck indoors, you are more likely to be deficient (see Box 5-4, "Vitamin D from Sunshine").

Without sun exposure, it can be difficult to obtain adequate vitamin D from food alone (see Box 5-5, "Getting Your Vitamin D"). Those at risk for vitamin D deficiency may want to consider supplements to reach the targets recommended by the Institute of Medicine (IOM). The IOM says people ages 70 and older should aim for a daily intake of vitamin D of 800 IU (International Units), 600 IU for those age 69 years and younger. But most older people, the IOM advises, do not need routine measurement of their blood levels of vitamin D.

Vitamin D Deficiency

It is clear that people with too little vitamin D are more likely to suffer cognitive impairment, even though the cause and effect in that connection are tough to untangle. In one study, the largest of its kind, older individuals deficient in vitamin D were significantly more likely to develop dementia and Alzheimer's over almost six years of follow-up than individuals with higher blood levels of the vitamin. Researchers characterized the results as "surprising" and said the association was twice as strong as anticipated.

They cautioned, however, that this kind of "prospective" study can't prove cause and effect; it is possible that vitamin D deficiency represents a consequence, rather than a cause, of cognitive deficits in elderly individuals.

Scientists reviewing the evidence on vitamin D and the brain reported that in 18 out of 25 cross-sectional observational studies, individuals with low vitamin D levels did more poorly on tests of cognitive functioning or displayed a higher frequency of dementia than individuals with higher blood levels of the vitamin. Similarly, four out of six prospective observational studies showed a higher risk of cognitive decline after a follow-up period of four to seven years in participants with lower vitamin D levels at baseline.

Recent research has even suggested that vitamin D helps clear beta-amyloid, the substance that forms the brain plaques associated with Alzheimer's disease. It may help prevent the degeneration of brain tissue by promoting the formation of neurons and maintaining the body's levels of calcium. It has also been proposed that vitamin D protects against age-related inflammatory changes in the brain's hippocampus.

Not So Fast

But the promising findings of observational studies of vitamin D have mostly failed to find support in more rigorous clinical trials, considered the "gold standard" of scientific research. A 2016 editorial in *JAMA Internal Medicine* put it this way: "The vitamin D story seems to be following the familiar pattern observed with antioxidant vitamins," such

BOX 5-4

Vitamin D from Sunshine

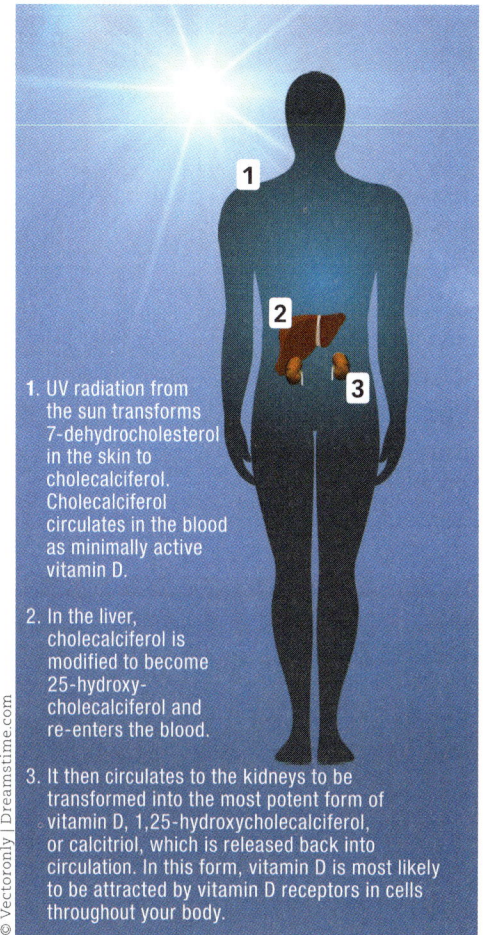

© Vectoronly | Dreamstime.com

1. UV radiation from the sun transforms 7-dehydrocholesterol in the skin to cholecalciferol. Cholecalciferol circulates in the blood as minimally active vitamin D.

2. In the liver, cholecalciferol is modified to become 25-hydroxy-cholecalciferol and re-enters the blood.

3. It then circulates to the kidneys to be transformed into the most potent form of vitamin D, 1,25-hydroxycholecalciferol, or calcitriol, which is released back into circulation. In this form, vitamin D is most likely to be attracted by vitamin D receptors in cells throughout your body.

BOX 5-5

Getting Your Vitamin D

Dietary sources of vitamin D are relatively scarce and include fortified milk, fortified brands of orange juice and breakfast cereal, and oily fish, such as salmon, mackerel, herring, and sardines. Your skin naturally makes vitamin D from cholesterol when exposed to ultraviolet light. Tufts vitamin D expert Bess Dawson-Hughes, MD, recommends getting a little sun—up to 15 minutes before applying sunscreen—when the season allows. "It's good to get a minimal amount of sun," she says. "It doesn't take a lot of sun to get vitamin D protection, without getting so much as to be toxic in terms of skin cancer."

In winter months when sunshine is scarce, she says, you may want to consider a vitamin D supplement. Dr. Dawson-Hughes warns against taking "extra" multivitamins to boost your vitamin D, which can mean getting too much vitamin A. Instead, she advises combining a vitamin D supplement containing 400 International Units (IU) with a multivitamin containing 400 IU.

BOX 5-6

Foods High in Antioxidant Vitamins

VITAMIN C	SERVING	MILLIGRAMS (MG)
Guava, raw	½ cup	188 mg
Red sweet pepper, raw	½ cup	142 mg
Kiwi fruit	1 medium	70 mg
Orange, raw	1 medium	70 mg
Orange juice	¾ cup	61-93 mg
Green pepper, sweet, raw	½ cup	60 mg
Grapefruit juice	¾ cup	50-70 mg
Strawberries, raw	½ cup	49 mg
Brussels sprouts, cooked	½ cup	48 mg
Cantaloupe	½ cup	47 mg
Broccoli, cooked	½ cup	37 mg

VITAMIN E	SERVING	MILLIGRAMS (MG)
Cereals, fortified, ready-to-eat	1 oz.	1.6-12.8 mg
Sunflower seeds, dry roasted	1 oz.	7.4 mg
Almonds	1 oz.	7.3 mg
Sunflower oil	1 Tbsp	5.6 mg
Safflower oil	1 Tbsp	4.6 mg
Hazelnuts (filberts)	1 oz.	4.3 mg
Mixed nuts, dry-roasted	1 oz.	3.1 mg
Turnip greens, frozen, cooked	½ cup	2.9 mg
Tomato paste	¼ cup	2.8 mg
Peanut butter	2 Tbsp	2.5 mg
Canola oil	1 Tbsp	2.4 mg
Avocado, raw	½ avocado	2.1 mg

BETA-CAROTENE (VITAMIN A EQUIVALENT)	SERVING	MICROGRAMS (MCG)
Carrot juice	¾ cup	1,692 mcg
Sweet potato with peel, baked	1 medium	1,096 mcg
Pumpkin, canned	½ cup	953 mcg
Carrots, cooked from fresh	½ cup	671 mcg
Spinach, cooked from frozen	½ cup	573 mcg
Kale, cooked from frozen	½ cup	478 mcg
Cantaloupe, raw	¼ medium	233 mcg
Red sweet pepper, cooked	½ cup	186 mcg

as vitamin E, beta-carotene, and vitamin C. In that pattern, the editorial noted, initial enthusiasm for supplementation, reinforced by observational studies "showing, essentially, that healthy people have higher vitamin levels," fails to be supported by subsequent randomized clinical trials or meta-analyses.

The bottom line? Consult with your healthcare professional if you think you might be at risk for deficiency. Taking a small vitamin D supplement—1,000 IU or less—won't hurt you, but you shouldn't count on those pills as your main brain defense.

Rethinking Antioxidants

By trapping compounds called "free radicals," antioxidants, such as vitamins C and E and beta-carotene, prevent oxidative damage to cells—including cells in the brain. You've probably read about the "miraculous" benefits of antioxidants in magazines and popular health books. Nutrition scientists now tend to think of these compounds not solely for their "antioxidant" capacity, however, and are cautious about claims that extra antioxidants in pill form will improve your health.

Most of the phytochemical nutrients, like flavonoids and anthocyanins, discussed in the previous chapter are also antioxidants. The health effects of these compounds go well beyond their ability to counter free radicals.

Antioxidants and Cognition

Since many of the foods high in antioxidants also seem to have brain benefits, such as fruits and vegetables (see Box 5-6, "Foods High in Antioxidant Vitamins"), scientists have explored whether supplements of these same compounds might have similar protective effects. To date, the results are mixed—certainly no reason to switch from fruits and vegetables to pills. And since the mechanisms of the protective effects of fruits and vegetables on the brain remain not fully explained, the only way to be sure to experience them is by consuming whole foods.

An exhaustive review of the evidence of how antioxidant nutrients affect cognitive performance narrowed 850 eligible studies down to the 10 best. The most convincing evidence, scientists concluded, involved blood levels of selenium and the intake of vitamins C, E, and carotenes, mostly from dietary sources. A decrease in selenium levels in the blood over nine years was associated with an accelerated decline in global cognition, attention, and psychomotor speed. People in the highest one-fifth of intake of vitamins C, E, and carotenes exhibited a slower rate of global cognitive decline over three years.

Other studies showing evidence of beneficial associations of higher dietary intake of vitamin E and flavonoids, as well as higher blood beta-carotene levels, were judged to be of lower quality. The review concluded, "There is a possibility for protective effects of antioxidant nutrients against decline in cognition in older people, although the supportive evidence is still limited."

Studying Vitamin Supplements

Another study reviewed a lengthy randomized trial of supplementation, involving more than 4,000 people. Those in the antioxidant supplement group received 120 milligrams of vitamin C, 6 milligrams of beta-carotene, 30 milligrams of vitamin E, 100 micrograms of selenium, and 20 milligrams of zinc daily. Five years later, participants underwent a battery of cognitive tests. Those who had been in the antioxidant group scored better in episodic memory (recollection of events that happened to you) than those who received a placebo; however, nonsmokers and those low in vitamin C at the beginning of the trial scored higher on verbal memory (recalling words from a list).

Most recently, a study specifically focused on supplements of vitamins C and E found an association between the extra vitamins and reduced risk of cognitive decline (see Box 5-7, "Antioxidant Vitamins Might Help Prevent Decline").

Vitamin E Against Alzheimer's

Other recent evidence indicates that extra vitamin E might slow the progression of Alzheimer's disease, but it doesn't mean healthy people should run out and buy vitamin E pills. A study of more than 600 mostly male veterans at 14 Veterans Affairs (VA) hospitals across the country compared a placebo with three treatments for patients with mild or moderate Alzheimer's: high-dose (2,000 IU daily) vitamin E supplements; a combination of vitamin E and memantine, a drug that's been shown to have modest benefits in moderate-to-severe Alzheimer's; and memantine alone. Only the vitamin E group saw any benefit, a small but statistically significant difference in tests of functional impairment over a period of more than two years. All three groups declined in their ability to perform tasks of daily living, but the vitamin E group declined the least.

The results, experts note, are specific to individuals already suffering with moderate-to-severe Alzheimer's disease and don't generalize to a healthy population. Other specific trials of vitamin E supplementation have failed to find a link between vitamin E supplements and risk of cognitive decline.

You may want to think twice about taking vitamin E supplements, which could have downsides. Two clinical trials have found an increased risk of hemorrhagic stroke in participants taking vitamin E (alpha-tocopherol). Two meta-analyses of randomized trials also have raised questions about the safety of large doses of supplemental vitamin E, including doses lower than the safe upper limit (UL) of 1,500 IU daily. These meta-analyses linked supplementation to small but statistically significant increases in all-cause mortality. Results from the large SELECT trial also showed that vitamin E supplements (400 IU/day) may harm adult men in the general population by increasing their risk of prostate cancer.

NEW FINDING   BOX 5-7

Antioxidant Vitamins Might Help Prevent Decline

Studies of antioxidant supplements as protection against cognitive decline and dementia are relatively few and have mostly been disappointing. But a new Canadian study might spark further research on these possible benefits. Researchers analyzed data on 5,269 participants, ages 65 and up, from the 11-year Canadian Study of Health and Aging, a study of dementia including three evaluation points. Self-reported use of vitamin E and vitamin C supplements at the study's start was compared with subsequent rates of cognitive impairment without dementia, Alzheimer's disease, and all-cause dementia. Compared with participants not taking the extra vitamins, risk of cognitive impairment was 23 percent lower, Alzheimer's was 40 percent lower, and all-cause dementia was 38 percent lower for those taking supplements. Results were similar when the vitamins were analyzed separately, and remained significant after adjusting for all other risk factors except for cognitive decline. Further investigations are needed to determine the supplements' value as a primary prevention strategy, researchers noted.

Annals of Pharmacotherapy, Oct. 4, 2016

Beta-Carotene Long-Term

Beta-carotene is converted by the body into vitamin A. Supplements of beta-carotene might have brain benefits, but only when taken for an extended period of time. Researchers reported that men who took 50-milligram supplements of beta-carotene every other day for an average of 18 years did significantly better on cognitive tests, especially those measuring verbal memory, than those taking a placebo. The benefit was the mental equivalent of being one year younger. But no similar protection against brain aging was observed in individuals given supplements for only a year.

As with vitamin E, however, there is a caution: Smokers should not take extra beta-carotene because of increased risk of lung cancer. Two well-designed clinical trials have reported that supplements of beta-carotene, alone or in combination with vitamin E supplements, increased the risk of lung cancer in smokers, compared to placebo.

Lutein and Zeaxanthin

Lutein and zeaxanthin, other carotenoid compounds found in leafy greens and other foods, form important pigments in the macula of the eye; supplements designed to reduce the risk of macular degeneration contain both. Lutein and zeaxanthin are the only carotenoids that cross the blood-retina barrier and accumulate in the human brain.

A small study compared macular pigments in 36 Alzheimer's patients and 33 healthy controls of the same age. The Alzheimer's patients were found to have significantly lower amounts of macular pigment and lower blood levels of lutein and zeaxanthin. They also had poorer vision and a higher incidence of macular degeneration.

Most recently, however, the same Age-Related Eye Disease Study (AREDS) that proved disappointing about fish oil pills also failed to find cognitive benefits from lutein and zeaxanthin. The same caveat about the study population applies to these conclusions, though, so scientists are continuing to look at these carotenoids.

Eat Your Nutrients

Unfortunately, science has yet to find any "magic bullet" in pill form that can safeguard your aging brain—even when testing nutrients that seem to have brain benefits when consumed from food. Taking a daily multivitamin won't hurt you, but an overall healthy diet is better for your brain than counting on "insurance" from a supplement. With advice from your healthcare professional, you might decide to supplement your dietary intake of vitamin B12 and/or vitamin D, which you could be falling short on as you age.

But the evidence simply is not strong enough to single out any specific nutrient supplement for brain benefits. As we'll see in the next chapter, the science behind most "supplements" touted specifically for cognition is, at best, even shakier.

PUTTING BRAIN SUPPLEMENT CLAIMS TO THE TEST

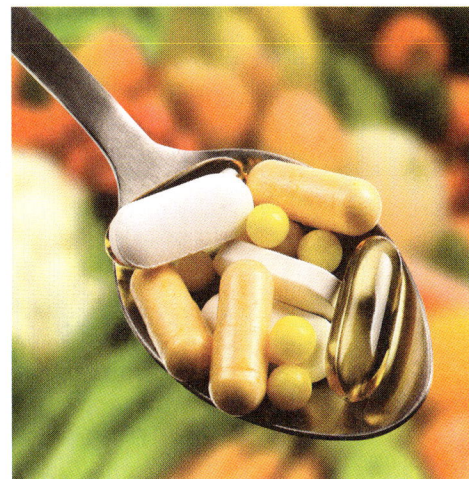

© Ronstik | Dreamstime.com

You can't watch the nightly news or open a magazine these days without seeing ads for brain-boosting nutritional supplements that claim to protect your memory or improve cognition. These range from mega-doses of vitamins your body does actually need in very small amounts to novel concoctions, such as Asian herbal remedies or proteins "originally found in jellyfish" (creatures that, ironically, don't even have brains). Do the claims for such products stand up to scientific scrutiny? While at least some evidence supports brain benefits for the nutrients we looked at in the last chapter, especially when obtained from food, other supplements sold for brain health lack this foundation in nutrition. Rather than providing extra vitamins, minerals, or essential fats that the body needs, these ingredients are marketed more like the magic elixirs of the old "medicine shows."

That in itself does not mean these "brain-boosting" pills are of no value, of course. In fact, scientists have reported some intriguing results about lesser-known nutrients. However, other studies largely debunk dietary supplements touted for brain benefits.

Be Regulatory Wise

Like all products sold as dietary supplements, "brain-boosting" supplements are regulated differently from foods or prescription drugs. Products that actually supplement what your body needs, such as extra calcium or vitamin D, are lumped in with herbal remedies that don't truly "supplement" a proven nutritional need. (No one needs extra ginseng, for example, and there is no evidence that you need any at all.)

While the U.S. Food and Drug Administration (FDA) has the power to ensure the safety of foods and medications and regulate health claims, dietary supplements fall under the 1994 Dietary Supplement Health and Education Act (DSHEA). Under DSHEA, the manufacturer is responsible for the accuracy and truthfulness of product claims, which must be submitted to the FDA within 30 days of use but are not verified by the government.

You've probably seen the disclaimer on product labels and ads complying with the rules of DSHEA: "This statement has not been evaluated by the Food and Drug Administration. This product is not intended to diagnose, treat, cure, or prevent any disease." Nonetheless, manufacturers can make carefully crafted promises—"structure-function claims" permitted under DSHEA—that their products, for example, "enhance mental sharpness and support long-term brain health" (not "prevent Alzheimer's disease").

What's in Those Pills?

When you buy "brain-boosting" supplements, you mostly have no guarantee of their purity, or even whether they actually contain the

BOX 6-1

Getting What You Pay for in the Supplement Aisle

If you decide to try an herbal remedy in hopes it will boost your brain, how can you be sure you're getting what you pay for? Look for products with the "USP Verified" seal of the United States Pharmacopeial Convention, an independent, nonprofit organization. Only products that have been voluntarily submitted to the USP and passed its testing can display the black-and-yellow seal. (Don't be fooled by labels that simply use the letters "USP," suggesting that the manufacturer claims to follow the organization's standards but doesn't submit products for testing.) Just a few nationwide brands, however, participate in the USP testing program. For a full list, see www.usp.org and click on "Verification Services" under "Dietary Supplements."

Another nonprofit, NSF International, www.nsf.org, focuses on products for athletes but also certifies some products such as multi-vitamins and fish oil. Two for-profit groups that test, rank, and review supplements are ConsumerLab, www.consumerlab.com, and LabDoor, www.labdoor.com.

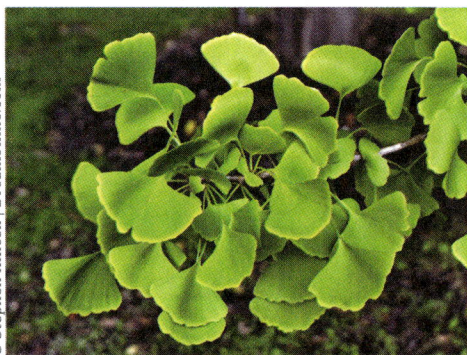

Ginkgo Biloba is extracted from the leaves of the plant.

© Stephen Kinosh | Dreamstime.com

ingredients listed on the label. Many consumers were shocked at news a few years ago that four out of five popular herbal remedies sold at some of the nation's leading retailers didn't contain *any* of the promised ingredients. DNA testing of store-brand products instead detected fillers—including wheat and legumes, which could pose risks for people with intolerances or allergies. For example, pills sold as ginkgo biloba, a Chinese plant touted for memory benefits, actually contained powdered radish, ground houseplants, and wheat.

Scientists at the University of Guelph in Canada reported that one-third of 44 herbal remedies tested contained no trace of the supposed main ingredient at all (see Box 6-1, "Getting What You Pay for in the Supplement Aisle").

You might even be getting unregulated pharmaceutical-grade drugs in your "brain-boosting" supplements. A recent study of supplements containing vinpocetine and picamilon sold in U.S. chain stores found that many deliver the same dose as that prescribed pharmacologically in other countries. Both are prescribed elsewhere as cerebrovascular drugs; vinpocetine is refined from an alkaloid found in the periwinkle plant, while picamilon is only produced synthetically. Neither has been approved as a prescription drug in the United States by the FDA, and both may have dangerous side effects for some patients. The study analyzed 23 brands of vinpocetine and 31 brands of picamilon supplements using ultra-high performance liquid chromatography to determine the accuracy of their labels. Only 26 percent of the vinpocetine labels were accurate in their dose data; others ranged from 0.3 to 32 milligrams (mg) per recommended daily dose (the pharmaceutical dose is 5 to 40 mg). On the other hand, six samples actually contained zero vinpocetine. The picamilon supplements ranged from 2.7 to 721.5 mg per dose; prescription doses range from 50 to 200 mg.

The Science on Herbal Supplements
The Latest on Ginkgo Biloba

Hope seems to spring eternal for ginkgo biloba, a Chinese herbal remedy derived from the leaves of the ginkgo tree. It's probably the best-known supplement promising brain benefits. Despite previous negative results from a large-scale clinical trial, new reviews of the evidence keep holding out possible benefits. A 2015 systematic review and meta-analysis involving a total of 2,561 participants concluded that 240 milligrams daily of ginkgo biloba stabilized or slowed decline in cognition, function, and behavior. A 2016 review also found potential benefits for patients with MCI or Alzheimer's (see Box 6-2, "Taking a Fresh Look at Ginkgo Biloba Evidence").

These somewhat positive findings stand in contrast to those of the Ginkgo Evaluation of Memory (GEM) study, a large and long-running clinical trial. GEM was a randomized, double-blind, placebo-controlled trial—the type considered the "gold standard" of medical research—involving 3,069 participants, ages 72 to 96, at six academic medical centers. Researchers reported no difference in the rate of total dementia or in the rate of Alzheimer's-type dementia between those given ginkgo and those administered a placebo. Participants already suffering from mild cognitive impairment saw no benefit from ginkgo biloba in preventing the progression to dementia. Subsequently, GEM also found that twice-daily doses of 120 milligrams of ginkgo extract worked no better than a placebo in slowing cognitive decline.

Those negative results were further supported by a French study testing 120 milligrams of ginkgo twice a day versus placebo among 2,854 patients, ages 70 and up. Participants were free of dementia, but had reported memory problems to their physicians. After five years of follow-up, 61 of those randomly assigned to ginkgo and 73 in the placebo group developed dementia—a difference scientists said was not statistically significant.

The bottom line? At best, further research is needed before recommending gingko supplements, which may have side effects, including gastrointestinal upset, allergic reactions, and increased bleeding risk.

Little Evidence for Ginseng and Grape-Seed Extract

Ginseng and grape-seed extract are also plant products popularly marketed for brain benefits, among other claims. These have not been as extensively studied as ginkgo, which means the evidence for any possible benefits is thin. A review by the National Center for Complementary and Integrative Health concluded there's not enough evidence to recommend these herbal remedies for protection against dementia and Alzheimer's disease.

Only a few high-quality clinical trials have been conducted on Asian ginseng in Alzheimer's disease, so the evidence pro or con is scant. According to the review, "Research results to date do not conclusively support health claims associated with the herb."

As for grape-seed extract, a few preliminary studies have looked at possible effects on the brain, but "there is currently insufficient evidence to determine if grape-seed extract is helpful in the prevention or treatment of cognitive decline or Alzheimer's disease." The Center is pursuing further research on grape-seed extract and brain disorders, as well as for possible heart benefits.

Other Brain Claims

The only way to know what you're getting in supplements sold for memory or "brain power" is close scrutiny of the Supplement Facts label. You might see other supplement ingredients with purported brain benefits, often sold in combination with the better-known ginkgo biloba. Few of these less-familiar ingredients have been studied extensively, and even those for which preliminary results seem somewhat promising should be considered, at best, unproven:

♦ Vinpocetine: Sometimes added to supplements containing ginkgo, vinpocetine is a synthetic compound made to resemble a substance found naturally in the periwinkle plant. It has been used in Europe to

NEW FINDING   BOX 6-2

Taking a Fresh Look at Ginkgo Biloba Evidence

Ginkgo biloba, an herbal remedy popularly sold for brain benefits, has largely failed to live up to such claims in rigorous clinical trials. But a recent review of 21 trials totaling 2,608 participants nevertheless found some positives for the traditional remedy. Compared with conventional medicine alone, ginkgo biboba in combination with conventional medicine was superior in improving Mini-Mental State Examination (MMSE) scores at 24 weeks for patients with Alzheimer's disease and mild cognitive impairment. The addition of ginkgo biloba was also associated with better scores on Activity of Daily Living tests among patients with Alzheimer's.

When compared with placebo or conventional medicine in individual trials, ginkgo biloba demonstrated similar but inconsistent findings; adverse events were mild. The researchers cautioned, however, that "the general methodological quality of included trials was moderate to poor." Due to limited sample size, they added, inconsistent findings and methodological quality of included trials, more research is warranted to confirm the effectiveness and safety of ginkgo biloba in treating mild cognitive impairment and Alzheimer's disease.

Current Topics in Medicinal Chemistry, 2016

protect against strokes because it's thought to increase blood flow to the brain. By extension, vinpocetine is also hypothesized to improve brain function. Studies of its effectiveness on healthy humans are rare and have been very small. In studies of older adults with memory problems associated with poor brain circulation or dementia-related disease, however, vinpocetine produced significantly more improvement than a placebo on tests of attention, concentration, and memory.

⬧ **Phosphatidylserine (PS):** A fat-like substance found naturally in cell membranes, especially in the brain, PS is extracted from soybeans and, like vinpocetine, often sold in combination with other memory-boosters. Promoters may boast that PS is the only such ingredient with a qualified health claim approved by the FDA; they are less likely to repeat the FDA's qualification that "there is little scientific evidence for this claim." Nonetheless, it's worth noting that a few small, short-term studies have shown promising results with PS in elderly subjects already suffering from memory problems. In one case, 100 milligrams of PS plus 80 milligrams of phosphatidic acid significantly improved memory, mood, and cognition in elderly subjects. Patients with Alzheimer's disease experienced a stabilizing effect on daily functioning.

⬧ **Huperzine A:** This moss extract is a Chinese herbal remedy thought to increase levels of the neurotransmitter acetylcholine in the brain. One review of the evidence in 10 trials in patients with Alzheimer's disease or vascular dementia concluded that Huperzine A could "significantly improve" cognitive scores. Those findings, however, do not mean that Huperzine A protects against cognitive decline in healthy individuals, as is claimed by some supplement formulations.

Doubts About Jellyfish Protein

Apoaequorin, a protein "originally found in jellyfish," as noted in TV commercials, has been the subject of only limited research. Those studies have mostly been done by scientists employed by the supplement maker and few have been published in peer-reviewed journals. In 2012, the FDA issued a warning letter to the company saying the product's claims crossed the line to being an "unapproved new drug." The agency also cited more than 1,000 "adverse events" related to the product, some of which required hospitalization.

In January 2017, the Federal Trade Commission (FTC) and New York Attorney General Eric Schneiderman filed suit against the supplement maker. Schneiderman called the marketing "a clear-cut fraud, from the label on the bottle to the ads airing across the country." However, according to the *New York Law Journal* website, the charges were dismissed in Federal court in September 2017.

Benefits of Curcumin

Could the compound that gives curry powder its distinctive orange color also help protect your brain? Curcumin (not to be confused with the spice called cumin) is the key component in turmeric, that colorful curry ingredient. Turmeric has been a common ingredient for thousands of years in traditional South Asian cooking and has been a popular compound in traditional medicine there. Also known as Indian saffron, turmeric is harvested for its roots (rhizomes), which look much like ginger (to which the plant is related) except for turmeric's vivid golden-orange color.

Only in the last decade or so has the curcumin found naturally in turmeric become the object of research attention in the Western scientific community, with more than 4,000 research articles published. As a result, even though evidence for curcumin's benefits remains preliminary, turmeric can now be found not only in well-stocked supermarkets but also in stores selling vitamins and other supplements. In supplement form, it may be labeled as either turmeric or curcumin or both.

People living in countries in which curry is a stable of the diet have much lower rates of Alzheimer's disease than people in the United States, leading scientists to suspect that curcumin could help mental functioning. In fact, a study of more than 1,000 non-demented elderly Asians found that those who reported consuming the most curry performed better on the Mini-Mental State Examination than those who consumed less of the spice.

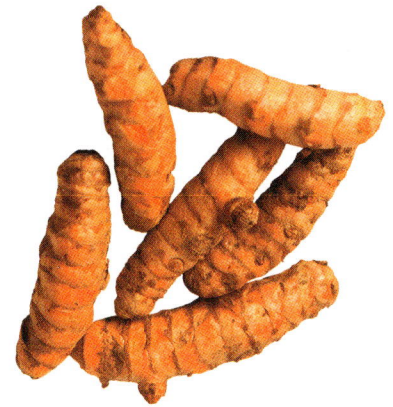

Tumeric is harvested for its roots, which look much like ginger.

Trials of Supplements

A pair of recent studies focused on supplements of curcumin, rather than relying on self-reported curry consumption and uncertain levels in the diet. One randomized, double-blind, placebo-controlled trial tested both the immediate and four-week effects of a 400-milligram curcumin supplement in 60 healthy adults ages 60 to 85. One hour after supplementation, those receiving curcumin showed significantly improved performance on tests of working memory and sustained attention. After four weeks of treatment, curcumin was associated with significant improvements in working memory and mood. No negative side effects were observed and, in fact, subjects given curcumin saw significant reductions in both LDL and total cholesterol levels.

The second study, published in 2016, was also a randomized, placebo-controlled, double-blind trial, lasting 12 months. Researchers investigated the ability of a curcumin formulation to prevent cognitive decline in a group of 96 community-dwelling older adults. Participants were randomly assigned to either a 1,500-milligram daily curcumin supplement or to a placebo. A battery of clinical and cognitive measures was administered at baseline and at six-month and 12-month follow-up assessments. The placebo group showed a decline in cognitive function at the six-month point that was not observed in the curcumin treatment group, resulting in a significant difference between the groups. No other differences were observed between the groups for all other clinical and cognitive measures, however. Researchers concluded, "Our findings suggest that further longitudinal assessment is required to investigate changes in cognitive outcome measures, ideally in conjunction with biological markers of neurodegeneration."

The Jury Is Still Out

Also in 2016, a comprehensive review of the evidence for benefits of curcumin against Alzheimer's disease noted that clinical trials mostly have not been able to demonstrate the expected benefits. But this has been broadly attributed to difficulties with absorption, bioavailability, and the timing and length of intervention. The review concluded that "there is significant evidence that curcumin can act on multiple pathways" in the development of Alzheimer's. Humans may be less responsive to curcumin than animals, however. Future studies, the review concluded, should concentrate on boosting the delivery of the compound and should include healthy community-dwelling older adults and those with subjective memory complaints, in longer-duration intervention studies.

Curcumin has antioxidant as well as anti-inflammatory properties, which may contribute for its apparent benefits.

Research at UCLA suggests that in addition to anti-inflammatory effects, curcumin helps the immune system remove beta-amyloid, the protein that forms damaging plaques in the brains of Alzheimer's patients. Curcumin also has a metal-chelation effect, binding to metals, such as copper, cadmium, and lead, that are toxic to nerve cells.

According to research in animals, curcumin could also promote the production of new brain cells (neurogenesis). These studies found that curcumin increases levels of brain derived neurotropic factor (BDNF), a molecule that encourages neurogenesis. BDNF also protects brain cells from damage and stimulates connections between brain cells.

It's possible that curcumin could be effective in countering depression and improving mood, because it seems to boost levels of the mood-enhancing neurotransmitters serotonin and dopamine. Much like the antidepressants called MAO inhibitors, curcumin blocks the enzymes responsible for breaking down serotonin and dopamine. Animal tests have shown that curcumin enhances the antidepressant effects of medications, like Prozac and Effexor.

Creatine for Muscles and Brains

An amino acid-like compound, creatine is used by athletes and body builders to boost muscle mass and improve performance in intense physical competitions, such as cycling or rowing. With sales of $400 million a year, creatine is one of the most popular dietary supplements. You can obtain creatine naturally in the diet through the consumption of high-protein foods, such as meat, fish, and eggs. The body also synthesizes creatine from amino acids.

Could extra creatine have benefits for the brain as well as your body's muscles? One review of the evidence concluded: "In relation to the brain, creatine has been shown to have antioxidant properties, reduce mental fatigue, protect the brain from neurotoxicity, and improve facets/components of neurological disorders like depression and bipolar disorder."

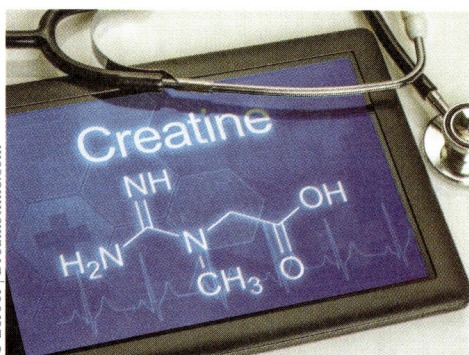

Creatine is an amino acid-like compound.

Supplements of creatine are generally believed to be safe and well tolerated by adults in amounts up to five grams per day; there's not enough evidence one way or the other about greater amounts.

The review added, "The combination of these benefits has made creatine a leading candidate in the fight against age-related diseases, such as Parkinson's disease, Huntington's disease, amyotrophic lateral sclerosis, long-term memory impairments associated with the progression of Alzheimer's disease, and stroke."

Improving Memory and Learning

In animal testing, mice and rats fed a diet enhanced with creatine displayed improved memory and learning ability. In studies of healthy humans, supplemental creatine significantly improved working memory and intelligence scores among vegetarians and vegans, who are likely to have low creatine intake from their diets.

Supplements of creatine also helped relieve the mental fatigue after an exam and improved mental performance of young men suffering from sleep deprivation. In a test of healthy non-vegetarians not subjected to any unusual stress, however, creatine supplementation did not improve scores on a variety of cognitive tests.

Alzheimer's and Creatine

Other studies have shown that patients with Alzheimer's disease have decreased activity of a creatine enzyme in key areas of the brain, compared with healthy people of the same age. It's possible that differences in this creatine enzyme contribute to the abnormal metabolism and neuron loss and dysfunction seen in Alzheimer's patients. The beta-amyloid plaques associated with Alzheimer's may inactivate or degrade this key creatine compound. Creatine also prevents oxidative damage, suggesting it might protect against beta-amyloid-induced oxidative stress in patients with Alzheimer's disease.

People suffering from age-related cognitive decline might also benefit. One study found improved performance on tests of verbal and spatial short- and long-term memory.

While more research is needed before recommending creatine as a tool against Alzheimer's and cognitive decline, the evidence to date is more encouraging than for other supplements more popularly touted as "brain boosters."

Mood and Behavior Supplements

In addition to memory and cognitive claims, many other supplements are marketed as beneficial for mood, depression, sleep quality, and "energy"—mental factors that affect behavior, which in turn can indirectly affect cognition. The evidence for their effectiveness is mixed, though some may be safe alternatives to prescription medications. You should also exercise caution when taking any of these supplements with prescription drugs; tell your health-care professional first.

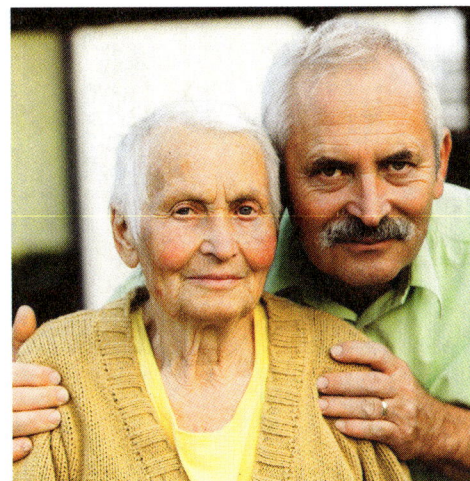

© Sandor Kacso | Dreamstime.com

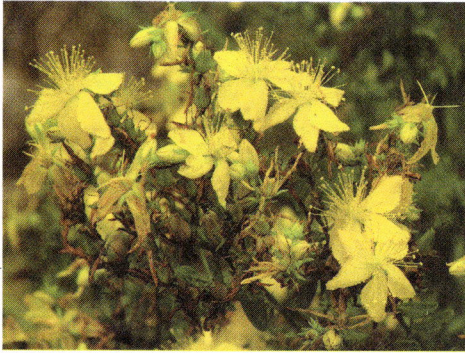
St. John's wort is a pretty flowering plant.

St. John's Wort

Derived from a flowering plant traditionally harvested on St. John's Day (June 24), St. John's wort is an option for short-term treatment of mild depression, according to clinical guidelines from the American College of Physicians-American Society of Internal Medicine. A review of the evidence about St. John's wort and major depression, published in the *Cochrane Database,* concluded that it was as effective as standard prescription antidepressants, with fewer side effects. The National Library of Medicine, however, cautions that although some studies have reported benefits for depression, others have not. One large study sponsored by NCCIH found that St. John's wort was no more effective than placebo in treating major depression of moderate severity.

Keep in mind, also, that St. John's wort has serious interactions with a long list of medications, including the blood thinner warfarin, so consult your physician before trying it. St. John's wort was also among the herbal products targeted by a recent investigation as frequently failing to actually contain the listed ingredient.

Green Tea

In chapter 4 we saw how tea might benefit memory and cognition. Green tea and green-tea extract also may combat depression. In one Japanese study, elderly participants who reported drinking four or more cups of green tea per day were 44 percent less likely to have symptoms of depression than those drinking one cup or less per day. A similar relationship was seen for green-tea consumption and risk of severe depression. The NCCIH adds, "Some evidence suggests that the use of green tea preparations improves mental alertness, most likely because of its caffeine content."

Valerian

An herbal remedy since ancient times, valerian is made from the root of the valerian, a flowering plant. It may be effective against insomnia, although the NCCIH advises, "There is not enough evidence from well-designed studies to confirm this." Moreover, "There is not enough scientific evidence to determine whether valerian works for other conditions, such as anxiety or depression."

Valerian does not relieve insomnia as fast as standard sleep medications, and continuous use for several days, even up to four weeks, may be needed before an effect is noticeable. Some studies have found that valerian doesn't improve insomnia any better than a placebo. Valerian should not be taken with alcohol or sedative medications.

Ephedra: Beware

An evergreen, shrub-like plant native to Central Asia and Mongolia, ephedra contains an active ingredient called ephedrine, which can powerfully stimulate the nervous system and heart. Besides its popular use in weight-loss supplements, ephedra has also been touted for "increased energy." But ephedra's risk of heart problems and stroke outweighs any benefits, according to the FDA, which in 2004 banned the sale of dietary supplements containing ephedra. The ban does not apply to traditional Chinese herbal remedies or to products like herbal teas regulated as conventional foods, so beware.

Energy Drinks' Downsides

You might also be tempted by the claims of so-called "energy drinks," which have soared in popularity in recent years. The FDA has investigated reports of adverse events tied to these beverages and cautions that these drinks are not alternatives to rest or sleep. The most common ingredients are caffeine, sugar, B vitamins, and amino acids. Although both caffeine and sugar can give you a short-term jolt, there are safer ways to obtain caffeine (as well as the healthy phytonutrients in coffee and tea), and sugar just adds calories.

Science vs. Snake Oil

Reading this chapter, you might have been surprised to learn how dubious are the claims for some of the most popularly promoted and sold supplements touted for brain benefits. On the other hand, supplements you may have never associated with brain power (or may never have heard of)—such as curcumin and creatine—seem to be the most promising. That's why it's important to keep up with the science of better brain power and stay skeptical about marketing claims, which are loosely regulated and may simply disguise what an earlier era would have called "snake oil."

In any case, none of the evidence for these brain-boosting supplements compares to the proven benefits of a healthy dietary pattern. Your best insurance against cognitive decline as you age can be found in your fridge and pantry—not in pill bottles—as well as in other elements of a healthy lifestyle, which we'll explore in the next chapter.

YOUR BRAINPOWER LIFESTYLE

I f exercise were a pill, experts say, everybody would take it. Although smart dietary choices can help protect your brain against age-related decline, the evidence that physical activity contributes to cognitive health is even stronger than the associations between nutrition and cognition. That's why the most important lifestyle change you can make for your brain happens between meals— increasing your level of physical activity, even if it's just brisk walking, gardening, or household chores (see Box 7-1, "Most-Active Seniors Show Less Cognitive Decline").

The evidence also shows that the sooner you start being active, the better. The CARDIA (Coronary Artery Risk Development in Young Adults) study reported that the more physically fit you are when you're younger, the more likely you are to keep your brain sharp as you age. Participants, originally ages 18 to 30, were tested for blood pressure, cholesterol levels, and other measures, and also walked at an increasingly fast pace on a treadmill until they couldn't continue. The young adults could stick with the treadmill test an average of 10 minutes. Each additional minute that a participant had been able to last on the original treadmill measurement was associated with the equivalent of about one year's less mental aging when they were given cognitive tests 25 years later.

But even if you were sedentary as a young adult, the study still had a glimmer of good news: The small group of participants who actually improved their fitness from the original treadmill testing scored better on the cognitive assessment than those whose fitness had declined or stayed the same.

In fact, other research has shown that even people already suffering from cognitive decline can benefit from becoming more physically active. A series of studies from North Carolina, Denmark, and Canada presented at the annual Alzheimer's conference found modest memory benefits when patients exercised 45 to 60 minutes three or four times a week. The workouts also improved quality of life for people in the early stages of Alzheimer's. One test using MRI scans showed increased blood flow in areas of the brain key to memory and cognition among patients who exercised—findings supported by cognitive testing. In people over 70 who exercised, tests of spinal fluid found a reduction in levels of the tau protein linked to Alzheimer's.

Up to Speed

Once you've started an exercise program with input from your healthcare professional, you can boost your brainpower even more by picking up the pace: More vigorous exercise is associated with greater cognitive protection. The National Walkers' Health Study, an analysis of data taken from almost 39,000 participants, found that a brisk pace has more benefits—even if the distance traveled is the same. Those

---

NEW FINDING BOX 7-1

Most-Active Seniors Show Less Cognitive Decline

Participants in the Northern Manhattan Study who reported being the most physically active were least likely to develop signs of cognitive decline—the equivalent of about 10 years of mental aging. The 876 participants were asked how long and how often they exercised during the previous two weeks. Most reported no exercise at all or only light exercise such as walking and yoga; only 10 percent reported moderate to high-intensity exercise, such as running or aerobics. An average of seven years later, each participant was given tests of memory and thinking skills and a brain MRI. Five years after that, they took the memory and thinking tests again. Among people with no initial signs of memory or thinking problems, those in the low-activity group showed greater declines on tests of how fast they could perform simple tasks and how many words they could recall from a list. The higher-activity 10 percent showed a difference equal to 10 years of aging—a disparity that remained after adjustment for other factors that could affect brain health.

Neurology, online March 23, 2016

reporting a pace slower than a 24-minute mile were at five-fold increased risk for mortality from dementia.

Upping walking speed even a little seemed to pay off, however: Those classified in the third-slowest category of walkers (about 15 to 17 minutes per mile) saw a significant reduction in their risk of dying prematurely compared to the slowest group. Looking specifically at dementia, each additional minute per mile in walking pace was associated with a 6.6 percent increased risk of mortality from Alzheimer's.

If walking doesn't interest you, consider dancing. Some research suggests that the combination of aerobic activity and concentrating on dance steps might pay brain dividends (see Box 7-2, "Dancing Might Have Special Brain Benefits").

Exercise and Your Hippocampus

The hippocampus, a key part of the inner brain involved in forming, storing, and processing memory, also benefits from a brisk walk. A study using data from the Exercise for Cognition and Everyday Living (EXCEL) trial of 86 women, ages 70 to 80, already suffering mild cognitive impairment compared the effects of exercise: One group engaged in a twice-weekly aerobic walking program, designed to increase in intensity to 70 percent to 80 percent of each individual's age-specific target heart rate. A second group was assigned to a resistance-training regimen, while a control group did only balance and stretching activities.

After six months, MRI scans found that those in the aerobics group saw a 5.6 percent increase in the size of the left hippocampus, a 2.5 percent increase in the right hippocampus, and a 4 percent increase in total hippocampus volume. Those in the other groups did not see significant increases in hippocampal volume. Researchers noted that the increases in hippocampal volume among the walkers with MCI were double that observed in a previous study of cognitively healthy older adults—suggesting brisk walking might be of most benefit to those at greatest risk for dementia.

Exercise and Genetic Risk

Exercise also may help protect people at higher genetic risk for Alzheimer's disease. Researchers who used PET scans to image the brains of people identified as carriers of APOE epsilon-4, a genetic risk factor for Alzheimer's, found that activity levels were inversely associated with amyloid plaque development in the brain. Among sedentary APOE epsilon-4 carriers, the scans showed greater buildup of the plaques associated with Alzheimer's. But the carriers who were physically active, meeting the American Heart Association guidelines for regular exercise, showed no more buildup of amyloid plaques than found in the brains of non-carriers. Those guidelines call for at least 150 minutes per week of moderate exercise or 75 minutes per week of vigorous exercise (or a combination of moderate and vigorous activity).

Dancing Might Have Special Brain Benefits

Consider adding dancing to your brain-healthy lifestyle. A new study suggests that learning a social dance, as in country dancing, might combine mind and body exercise in a way that's even more beneficial to the brain than walking. Researchers recruited 174 healthy but mostly sedentary people in their 60s and 70s for aerobic fitness and cognitive tests, along with MRI scans. The volunteers were then randomly split into three activity groups: stretching and balancing three times a week, brisk walking three times a week, or learning to dance. The dance group practiced increasingly complex choreography for an hour three times a week. After six months, participants were tested again. Most, especially the oldest volunteers, showed signs of degeneration in the brain's white matter. Those in the dance group, however, actually had denser white matter in the fornix, an area of the brain important to memory and processing speed. The changes were not reflected in cognitive testing, which mostly improved across the board; researchers said that suggests a time lag between structural brain changes and effects on thinking and memory. It's possible, they added, that the combined cognitive and physical activity of learning to dance could help delay such decline even further.

Frontiers in Aging Neuroscience, April 2017

BOX 7-3

How Much Activity?

The most up-to-date recommendations for adult physical activity come from the Physical Activity Guidelines for Americans, www.health.gov/PAGuidelines. For adults, the guidelines emphasize that everyone should avoid inactivity. Some physical activity is better than none, and adults who participate in any amount gain some health benefits. Specific guidelines for adults include:

- Do at least 150 minutes (2 hours and 30 minutes) a week of moderate-intensity, or 75 minutes (1 hour and 15 minutes) a week of vigorous-intensity aerobic physical activity, or an equivalent combination. Aerobic activity should be performed in episodes of at least 10 minutes; preferably, it should be spread throughout the week.

- For additional, more extensive health benefits, increase aerobic physical activity to 300 minutes (5 hours) a week of moderate intensity, or 150 minutes a week of vigorous intensity, or an equivalent combination.

- You should also do muscle-strengthening activities that are moderate or high intensity and involve all major muscle groups on two or more days a week.

How Active—Really?

Most studies of physical activity and cognition, however, suffer from a reliance on participants' self-reported activity levels. How can scientists be sure that subjects are really as active (or sedentary) as they say they are? Researchers at Rush University Medical Center sought to overcome that challenge using a wrist device called an actigraph. The device recorded movement of all kinds for 10 days at the start of the study to determine participants' average activity levels. The 716 participants, average age 82, were initially free of cognitive impairment.

Over the next four years, 71 of the study group developed Alzheimer's. Those in the bottom 10 percent of total physical activity were twice as likely to develop the disease as the most active 10 percent.

What About Strength Training?

Exercise guidelines recommend that, along with aerobic activity such as brisk walking, older people to engage in strength training, such as lifting weights (see Box 7-3, "How Much Activity?"). To find out whether strength training is also good for the brain, University of British Columbia scientists conducted a six-month randomized trial of 86 women, ages 70 to 80, who suffered from mild cognitive impairment. Those assigned to resistance training using machines and free weights significantly improved their scores on memory tests. The study compared resistance training versus aerobic exercise (an outdoor walking program) and a control group that did only balance and stretching activities. The aerobic group got fitter but saw no memory benefits.

In MRI scans of 22 participants, those in the weight-lifting group also saw significant functional changes in areas of the brain associated with cognition and memory, along with improving their test scores.

Brain Effects of Exercise
Activity and Plasticity

In chapter 1, we looked at recent discoveries about the brain's plasticity. Scientists formerly thought that age-related cognitive and brain changes were inevitable, and that the adult brain couldn't grow new neurons. Now we know that even adults can increase their number of neurons and the connections between them. Not surprisingly, physical activity helps this process, and seems to be one of the ways in which activity benefits the brain.

A University of Illinois study showed that as little as three hours a week of brisk walking can stimulate the brain's neurons. The research involved 59 healthy but sedentary volunteers, ages 60 to 79, who participated in a six-month randomized clinical trial. Half did aerobic exercises such as brisk walking, while a control group did only non-aerobic stretching and toning exercises. Researchers compared high-resolution MRI brain scans before and at the end of the exercise program. Those in the aerobic exercise group showed significant increases in brain volume, while those in the control group did not. The greatest gains from aerobic exercise were associated with the prefrontal and temporal cortices of the brain—areas responsible for memory and information processing that are especially prone to age-related deterioration.

Exercise vs. Atrophy and Shrinkage

Staying active also seems to correlate with reduced levels of brain atrophy and shrinkage (See Box 7-4, "Exercise, Activity Linked to More Grey Matter"). A University of Kansas study found that people with early Alzheimer's disease who did best on a treadmill test were also less prone to the brain atrophy associated with the disease. The study used the treadmill to measure peak oxygen consumption—a gauge of cardiorespiratory fitness—along with MRI scans to view the brains of 57 patients with early Alzheimer's and a control group of 64 people free of dementia. After controlling for age, higher peak oxygen consumption was associated with greater whole-brain volume. People with early Alzheimer's disease who were less physically fit had four times more brain shrinkage compared to normal older adults than people who were more physically fit.

Blood Flow and the Brain

We've already seen how closely the heart and brain are connected. By increasing blood flow to the brain, much as physical activity can improve cardiovascular health, being active might similar benefit your brain. In particular, in this way physical activity could reduce the risk for vascular dementia—the slow, progressive thief of memory and cognitive function associated with impaired blood circulation in the brain.

In an Italian study, regular, non-strenuous physical activity substantially reduced the risk of vascular dementia. Over a four-year span, participants who engaged the most regularly in moderate activity retained the most cognitive function. Regular walking was associated with a 73 percent risk reduction for vascular dementia.

Other studies have shown that burning as little as an extra 100 daily calories can be enough to move you out of the highest-risk, most sedentary population (see Box 7-5, "Mission: Burn 100 Calories").

Patients with cardiovascular health concerns also seem to show brain benefits from exercise. In the Women's Antioxidant Cardiovascular Study, for example, the equivalent of a daily, brisk, 30-minute walk was associated with lower risk of cognitive impairment. As activity levels increased, the rate of cognitive decline decreased. The study followed 2,809 women, average age about 73, who had either prevalent vascular disease or three or more coronary risk factors.

NEW FINDING　　　　　BOX 7-4

Exercise, Activity Linked to More Grey Matter

Here's more evidence that staying active as you age boosts your brain—specifically, grey matter in brain regions typically affected most by Alzheimer's. A study looked at data on almost 900 men and women, at least age 65 initially, who had complete medical and cognitive tests, answered questionnaires about their physical activity, and underwent MRI brain scans. From the questionnaires, researchers estimated how many weekly calories participants expended in exercise as well as activities such as gardening and dancing. After five years, the most active one-quarter of participants had significantly more grey matter in parts of the brain associated with memory and higher-level thinking, compared with their most sedentary peers. This difference was observed regardless of cognitive status. For participants who were cognitively normal at the time of the initial scan, the volume of grey matter in those areas of the brain was associated with subsequent risk of developing mild or severe cognitive impairment: Greater gray-matter volume predicted lower risk. Even among those initially diagnosed with dementia or mild cognitive impairment, the extent of brain atrophy was less in the high-activity group.

Journal of Alzheimer's Disease, Vol. 52 #2, 2016

BOX 7-5

Mission: Burn 100 Calories

Engaging in enough daily physical activity to burn about 100 calories can be the difference between a high-risk sedentary lifestyle and being "moderately inactive." Of course, you'll want to aim for a greater level of activity over time, but just getting going can pay big dividends. Here are examples of activities that burn about 100 calories, depending on your weight, in about 20 minutes:

- Walk briskly
- Gardening
- Lawn mowing with a power mower
- Play tennis doubles
- Rake leaves
- Roller-skate
- Shoot some baskets
- Wash and wax a large car

Can't spare 20 minutes? These more strenuous activities burn about 100 calories in 15 minutes:

- Box
- Dance fast
- Hike
- Ice-skate
- Lift weights
- Mow the lawn with a push mower
- Split wood
- Tread water
- Walk uphill
- Work out on a stair-climber

Cortisol Levels May Affect Alzheimer's Risk

A new review links poor sleep quality and diet to the early accumulation of the plaques associated with Alzheimer's disease. Part of the reason may involve cortisol, a hormone manufactured by the body that plays a role in regulating many core functions, including sleep. Cortisol levels naturally rise and fall with day and night. But diets characterized by high intakes of refined sugars, salt, animal fats and animal proteins, and by low intakes of fruits and vegetables, can perturb the circadian levels of cortisol, leading to poor sleep quality. The researchers noted several specific foods and nutrients that might be linked to cortisol regulation:

- Flaxseed has been reported to reduce responses to stress and cortisol levels.

- Phosphatidylserine (PS), a fat-like substance found naturally in cell membranes, especially in the brain, is extracted from soybeans and sold as a "memory-boosting" supplement.

- Magnesium deficiency is strongly correlated with insomnia.

- Potassium is important for adequate sleep duration.

- Sleep deprivation can cause a decrease of creatine in the brain, negatively affecting cognition and mood.

Advances in Nutrition, July 2016

Sleep and Brain Power

Getting a good night's sleep is important for a healthy brain, too. Findings from several studies suggest sleeping too little or too much, abnormal breathing during sleep, and excessive daytime sleepiness are significantly associated with cognitive impairment. Your diet could also be a factor in this sleep-cognition connection (see Box 7-6, "Cortisol Levels May Affect Alzheimer's Risk").

The importance of sleep doesn't mean napping the day away. Like Goldilocks, your brain seems to demand an amount of sleep that's neither too little nor too much, but just right. That "just right" amount for most people seems to be about seven hours of sleep, give or take an hour or so.

Evidence for this seven-hour sweet spot comes from the large, long-running Nurses' Health Study. Among more than 15,000 participants ages 70 and older, sleep quality was linked to cognitive health. After an initial cognitive examination, the women were followed for up to six years, including recording sleep duration and cognitive assessments. A subset of 468 women also had blood tests for the beta-amyloid compound associated with Alzheimer's disease. Compared to the women who slept about seven hours per night, those who slept two hours more or two hours less than seven hours performed worse on cognitive tests. Those sleeping five hours or less and nine hours or more also had beta-amyloid blood markers that predicted a greater risk of cognitive decline and dementia. Overall, abnormal sleep duration was cognitively equivalent to aging by two years.

In another long-term study, the French Three-City Study, which followed nearly 4,900 non-demented participants age 65 and older for up to eight years, excessive daytime sleepiness was associated with an increased risk of cognitive decline.

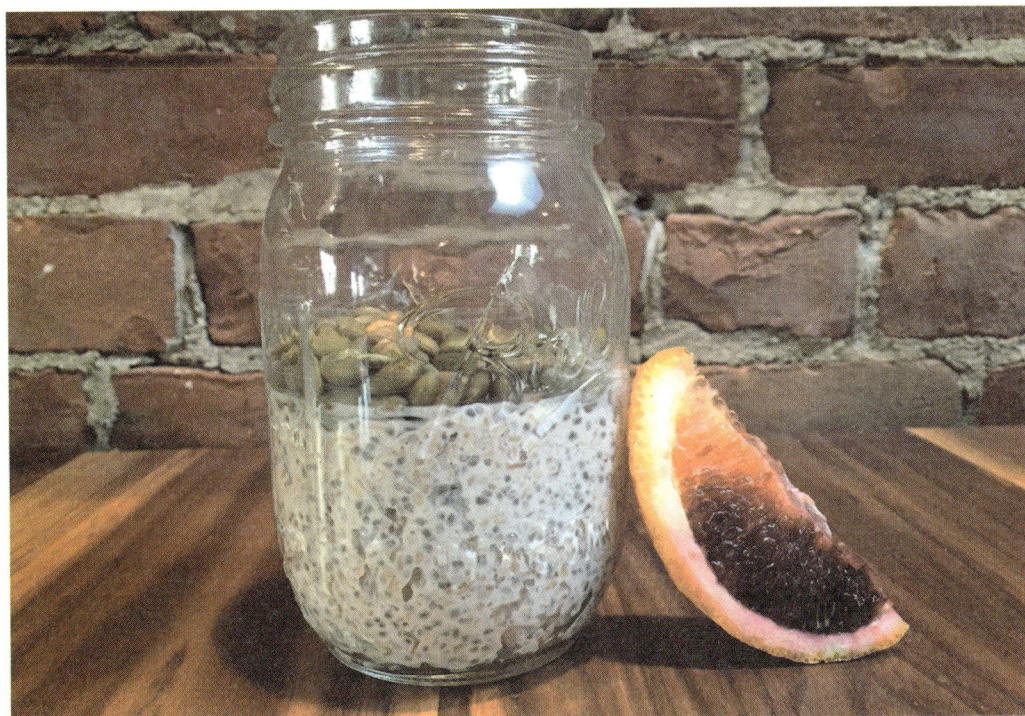

Cardamom and Orange Overnight Oats

Ingredients

½ cup plain Greek yogurt

1 cup rolled oats

1 cup unsweetened almond or coconut milk fortified with vitamin B-12

2 Tbsp chia seeds

1 Tbsp maple syrup

1 tsp orange zest

¼ tsp cardamom

¼ Tbsp ground cinnamon

1 Tbsp pumpkin seeds for garnish

Orange slices for garnish

Steps

1. In a Mason jar, mix yogurt, oats, milk, chia seeds, maple syrup, orange zest, cardamom, and cinnamon. Add the top to the Mason jar and shake.
2. Leave in the fridge overnight.
3. Top with pumpkin seeds and orange slices or other fruit.

Yield: 2 servings

Per serving: 301 calories, 8g total fat, 1g saturated fat, 16g protein, 43g carbs, 8g fiber, 9mg cholesterol, 123mg sodium

Source: Oldways Whole Grains Council, www.wholegrainscouncil.org

Roasted Salmon with North African Herb Sauce

Ingredients

- ¼ cup chopped fresh parsley
- ¼ cup chopped fresh cilantro (or more parsley)
- 2 medium cloves garlic, minced
- 1 tsp paprika
- 1 tsp ground cumin
- Pinch of ground red pepper (cayenne)
- ⅛ tsp salt, or to taste
- Pepper to taste
- ¼ cup nonfat plain yogurt
- 2 Tbsp lemon juice, plus wedges for serving
- 1 Tbsp vegetable oil
- 1 ⅛ lb salmon fillet (1 lb without skin), cut into 4 portions

Steps

1. Stir together parsley, cilantro, garlic, paprika, cumin, ground red pepper, salt, and pepper in small bowl. Add yogurt, lemon juice, and oil; mix well. Reserve ⅓ cup to serve as sauce; set aside, covered, in the refrigerator.
2. Place salmon pieces on plate. Rub remaining parsley mixture over fish. Cover and marinate in the refrigerator at least 20 minutes or up to 1 hour. Discard any used marinade.
3. Meanwhile, preheat oven to 400°F. Line a small baking sheet or baking pan with aluminum foil. Coat foil with cooking spray.
4. Transfer fish to prepared baking sheet. Bake until fish flesh is opaque and begins to flake, 12 to 20 minutes, depending on thickness. To estimate cooking time, use the rule of 10 minutes per inch of thickness. Serve with lemon wedges and reserved sauce.

Yield: 4 (3-oz fish) servings and ⅓ cup sauce
Per serving: 230 calories, 12g total fat, 2g saturated fat, 27g protein, 3g carbs, 1g fiber, 70mg cholesterol, 140mg sodium

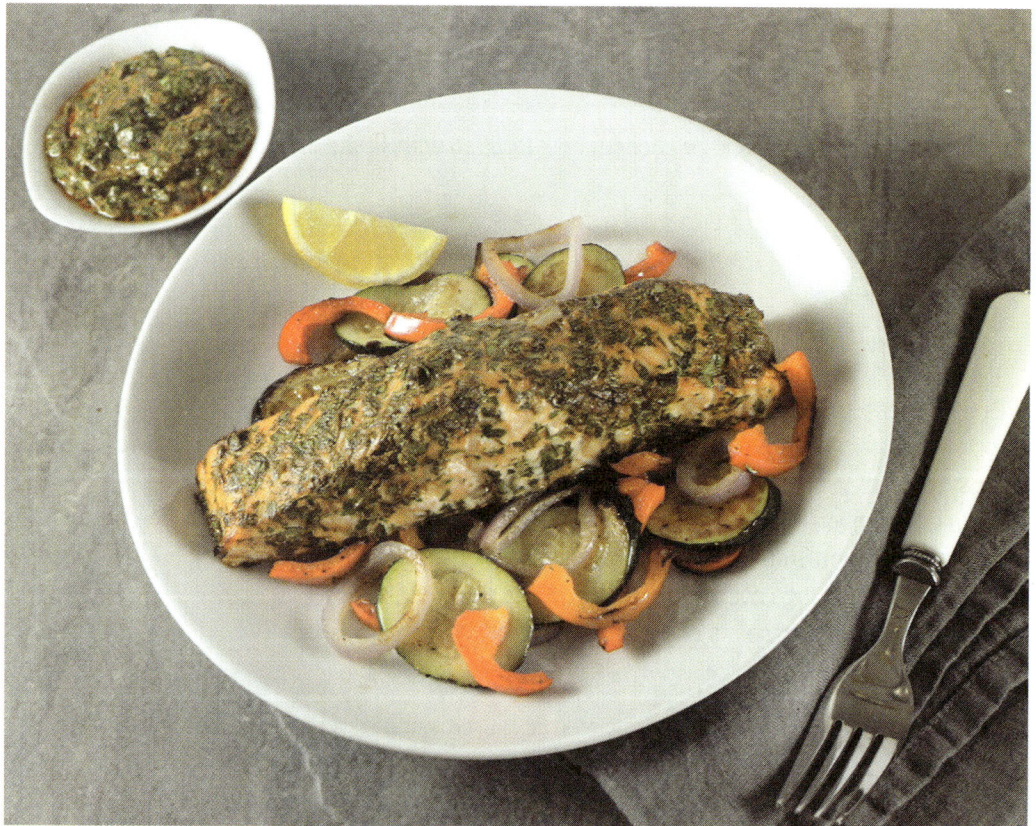

Mediterranean Kabobs

Ingredients

For marinade:

2 Tbsp olive oil

1 Tbsp garlic, minced (about 2 to 3 cloves)

2 Tbsp lemon juice

1 Tbsp fresh parsley, rinsed, dried, and chopped (or 1 tsp dried)

½ tsp salt

For kabobs:

6 oz top sirloin or other beef steak cubes (12 cubes)

6 oz boneless, skinless chicken breast, cut into ¾-inch cubes (12 cubes)

1 large white onion, cut into ¾-inch squares (12 pieces)

12 cherry tomatoes, rinsed

1 (4 oz) red bell pepper, rinsed and cut into ¾-inch squares (12 squares)

12 wooden or metal skewers, each 6 inches long (if wood, soak them in warm water for 5 to 10 minutes to prevent burning)

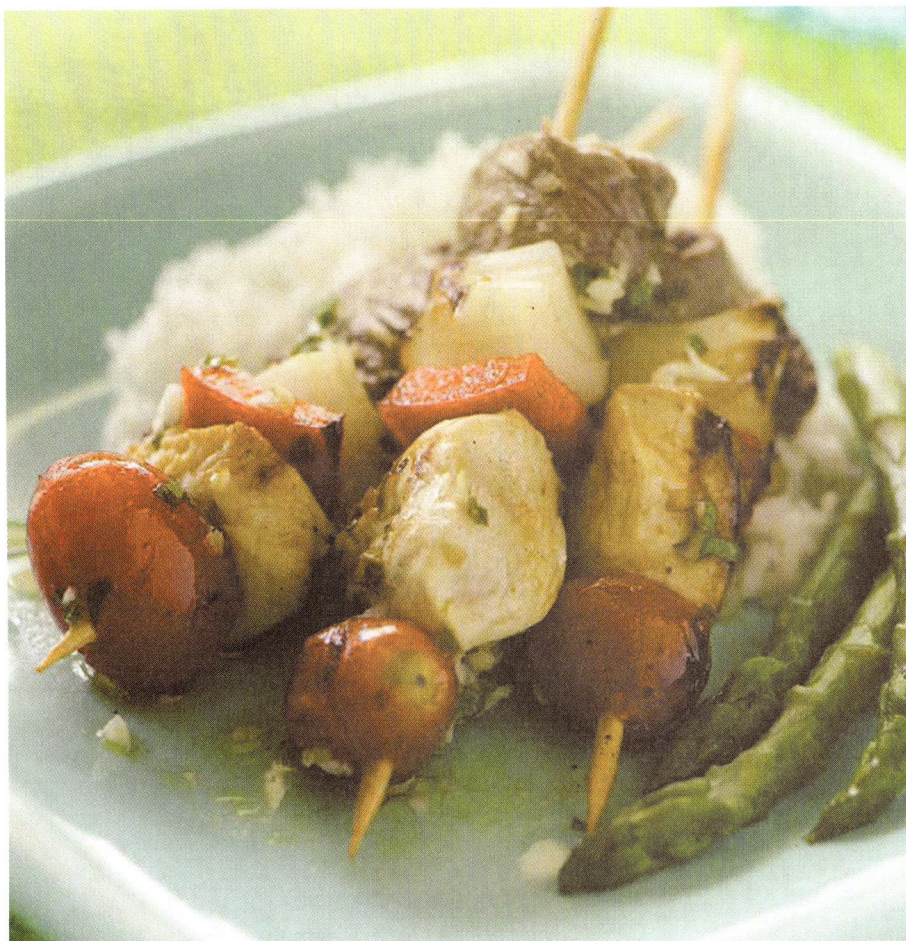

Steps

1. Preheat grill pan or oven broiler (with the rack 3 inches from heat source) on high temperature.
2. Combine ingredients for marinade, and divide between two bowls (one bowl to marinate the raw meat and one bowl for cooking and serving).
3. Mix the beef, chicken, onion, tomatoes, and red pepper cubes in one bowl of the marinade and let sit. After 5 minutes, discard remaining marinade.
4. Place one piece of beef, chicken, tomato, onion, and red pepper on each of the 12 skewers.
5. Grill or broil on each of the four sides for 2 to 3 minutes or until completely cooked (to a minimum internal temperature of 145°F for beef and 165°F for chicken). Spoon most of the second half of the marinade over the kabobs while cooking.
6. Serve three skewers per serving. Drizzle the remaining marinade on top of each kabob before serving (use only the marinade that did not touch the raw meat or chicken).

Yield: 4 (3 skewers) servings

Per serving: 202 calories, 11g total fat, 2g saturated fat, 18g protein, 9g carbs, 2g fiber, 40mg cholesterol, 333mg sodium

Source: National Heart, Lung & Blood Institute

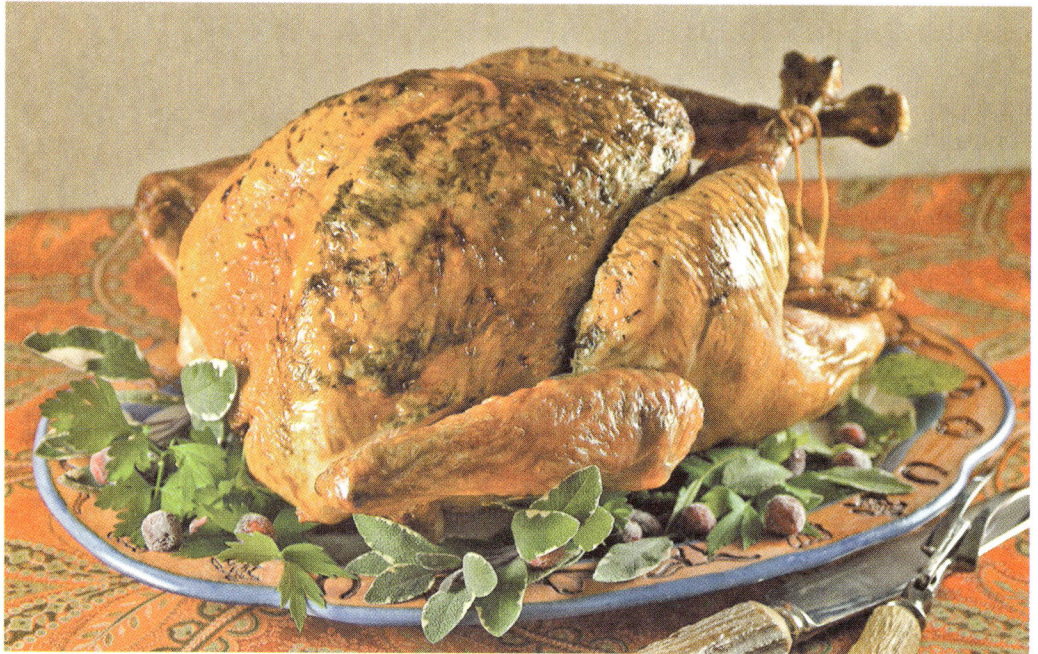

Herb-Roasted Turkey

Lean turkey is a brain-healthy choice any time of the year, though this recipe also shows you can eat right even at the holidays; use leftovers on whole-grain bread with lettuce and tomato for lunch.

Ingredients

3 Tbsp chopped fresh parsley

2 Tbsp chopped fresh rosemary

1 Tbsp chopped fresh thyme leaves

2 cloves garlic, minced

1 tsp lemon zest

¼ tsp salt

¼ tsp pepper

2 Tbsp olive oil

1 (12-to 14-lb.) turkey, fresh or thawed

2 medium onions, peeled and quartered

2 ½ cups Giblet Broth (recipe follows)

½ cup fortified wine, such as Madiera, Port, or Marsala, or dry white wine, apple cider, or pomegranate juice

2 Tbsp cornstarch mixed with ¼ cup water

Steps

1. Set oven rack on lowest shelf of oven; preheat to 325ºF. Coat a wire roasting rack, preferably a v-shaped rack, with cooking spray. Set rack in roasting pan.

2. Mix parsley, rosemary, thyme, garlic, lemon zest, salt, pepper, and oil in small bowl. Place turkey on cutting board. Remove giblets and neck from cavity and reserve for Giblet Broth. Reserve liver for another use. Rinse turkey inside and out with cold water. Pat dry with paper towels. Separate skin from breast meat and upper portion of thigh with your fingers, taking care not to pierce skin. Smear herb mixture between skin and flesh over breast meat and upper thigh. Stuff cavities with onion quarters. Tuck wing tips behind back and tie drumsticks together with kitchen twine. Set turkey, breast side up, on prepared rack. Tent loosely with aluminum foil.

3. Roast turkey 2 hours. Remove foil and continue roasting until meat thermometer registers 165 to 170ºF when inserted in thickest part of breast and 175-180ºF in thickest part of thigh away from bone, 1 to 1 ¾ hours. (Check temperature in both thigh and breast.)

4. While turkey roasts, make Giblet Broth (if you have not made it in advance).

5. Transfer turkey to large clean cutting board. Cover loosely with foil and let rest at least 20 minutes before carving. (While turkey rests you can heat side dishes.) Pour roasting

pan drippings into fat separator or glass measuring cup. Place in freezer to hasten separation of fat from lean drippings. Meanwhile, set roasting pan over 2 burners. Pour in wine (or cider or juice). Bring to a simmer over medium-high heat, stirring to scrape up brown bits. Simmer 1 to 2 minutes to intensify flavor. Pass through a strainer into medium saucepan. Add Giblet Broth and bring to a simmer. Simmer several minutes. Skim fat from the drippings you have placed in freezer (see Tip); stir into sauce. Stir cornstarch mixture; gradually add to simmering sauce, whisking constantly, until lightly thickened and glossy.

6. Remove twine from turkey. Carve turkey, discarding skin, and serve.

Giblet Broth

1. You can make the broth up to 2 days ahead and store it, covered, in the refrigerator. Alternatively, simmer the broth while the turkey roasts.

2. Heat 1 Tbsp canola oil in heavy 4- to 6-qt pan over medium-high heat. Pat turkey neck and giblets dry. Add to pan and cook, turning from time to time, until browned, 4 to 5 minutes. Transfer to a plate. Add 1 coarsely chopped onion, 2 coarsely chopped carrots; cook, stirring often, until browned, 4 to 6 minutes. Add 1 (32-oz) carton low-sodium chicken broth, 1 cup water, 1 rib celery (cut into several pieces), 4 cloves peeled garlic, 1 tsp black peppercorns, ½ tsp dried thyme leaves, and 1 bay leaf. Bring to a simmer. Skim froth. Reduce heat to low, partially cover and simmer 1 hour. Pour broth through a fine strainer into a medium bowl, pressing on solids to extract maximum flavor. Blot any fat from surface with paper towel. (If broth doesn't measure 2 ½ cups, add water.)

Yield: about 2 ½ cups gravy and enough turkey to serve 10, with leftovers.
Per (3 oz) serving of skinless white meat, before gravy: 150 calories, 4.5G total fat, 1g saturated fat, 25g protein, 0g carbs, 0g fiber, 60mg cholesterol, 105mg sodium
Per ¼ cup serving of gravy: 45 calories, 1.5G total fat, 0g saturated fat, 1g protein, 3g carbs, 0g fiber, 0mg cholesterol, 30mg sodium

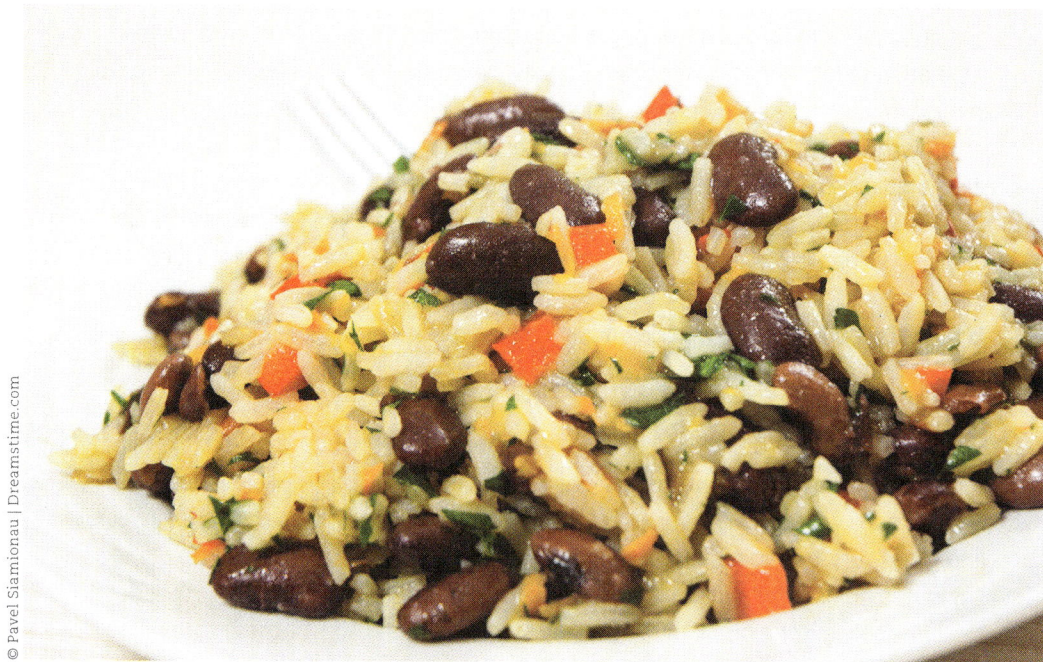

© Pavel Siamionau | Dreamstime.com

Vegetarian Red Beans and Rice

Ingredients

1 Tbsp olive oil

1 cup onion, cut into ½-inch pieces

1 cup green bell pepper, rinsed and diced

1 Tbsp garlic, minced or pressed (about 2 to 3 cloves)

1 ½ tsp ground cumin

1 ½ tsp dried oregano

1 can (14 ½ oz) low-sodium chicken broth or vegetable broth

½ cup instant brown rice, uncooked

2 cans (15 oz each) low-sodium red kidney beans, drained and rinsed

Steps

1. Heat oil in a 12-inch sauté pan over medium heat. Cook onion, stirring occasionally, for 5 minutes, until pieces begin to soften, but not brown.
2. Meanwhile, dice green pepper into pieces about ¼ inch in size. Add green pepper to cooking onion. Cover. Cook for 5 minutes, stirring occasionally.
3. While the green pepper and onion cook, mince the garlic. Add garlic, cumin, and oregano to the sauté pan. Cook and stir for 1 minute.
4. Add broth and rice to the sauté pan with green pepper and onion. Stir well, cover, and simmer for 10 minutes.
5. Meanwhile, drain beans and rinse thoroughly.
6. Add beans to sauté pan. Stir well. Cover. Simmer for 5 minutes to heat beans and blend flavors.

Yield: 4 servings (2 cups beans and rice)

Per serving: 344 calories, 5g total fat, 1g saturated fat, 18g protein, 57g carbs, 9g fiber, 2mg cholesterol, 331mg sodium

Source: National Heart, Lung, And Blood Institute

Warm Spiced Sweet Potato Salad With Spinach

Ingredients

⅓ cup thinly sliced red onion

3 Tbsp sliced almonds

1 lb sweet potatoes (1 large or 2 small),
   peeled and cut into ¾-inch chunks
   (2 ¾ cups)

¼ cup fresh orange juice

4 tsp lemon juice

½ tsp honey

½ tsp minced garlic (1 small clove)

½ tsp ground cinnamon

½ tsp ground ginger

½ tsp turmeric

½ tsp salt, or to taste

⅛ tsp pepper

2 Tbsp extra-virgin olive oil

4 cups baby spinach, washed and dried

Steps

1. Place onion in a medium bowl and cover with ice water. Let soak for 10 to 15 minutes.

2. Place almonds in microwave-safe bowl and microwave at High 1 to 2 minutes, or until fragrant and lightly toasted. (Alternatively, spread almonds in small baking pan; toast in 350° oven 10 to 15 minutes.) Let cool.

3. Meanwhile, place sweet potatoes in a large saucepan. Cover with water and bring to a simmer. Reduce heat to medium-low, cover and cook 5 to 7 minutes or just until tender but still firm. Drain.

4. While sweet potatoes are cooking, whisk orange juice, lemon juice, honey, garlic, cinnamon, ginger, turmeric, salt, and pepper in large bowl. Whisk in oil. Reserve 3 Tbsp of this dressing for spinach.

5. Add hot sweet potatoes to dressing in bowl. Drain onions and add to sweet potatoes; toss gently with rubber spatula to mix. Toss spinach with reserved 3 Tbsp dressing in a large bowl. Mound spinach on 4 plates. Top with sweet potato salad and sprinkle with toasted almonds. Serve warm.

Yield: 4 servings (¾ cup sweet potato salad and 1 cup spinach salad).
Per serving: 210 calories, 9g total fat, 1g saturated fat, 3g protein, 33g carbs, 5g fiber, 0mg cholesterol, 220mg sodium

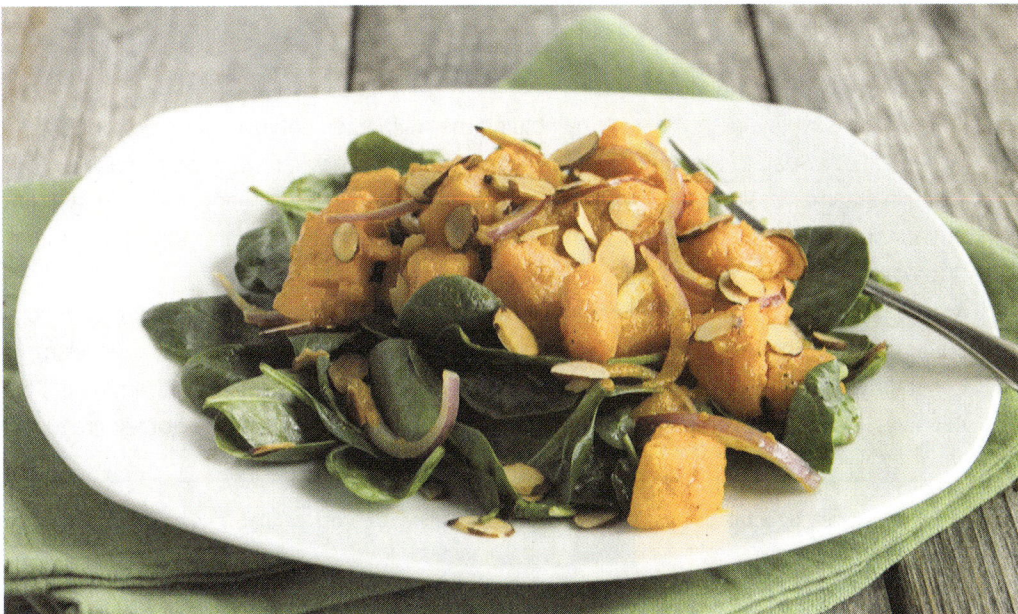

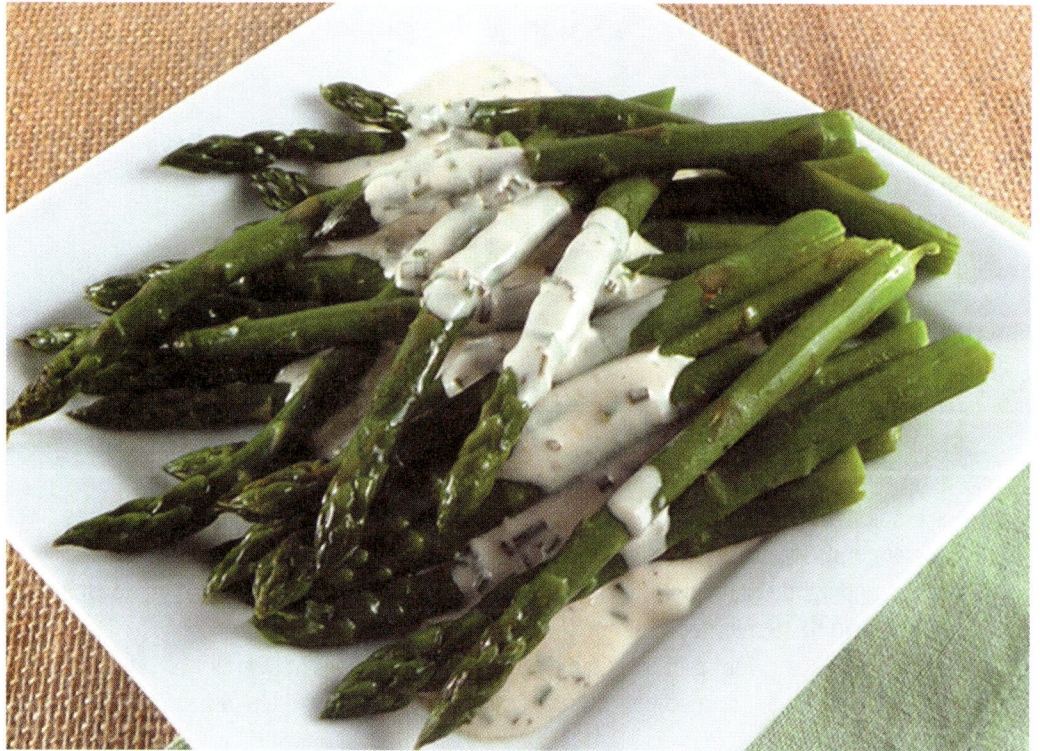

Asparagus With Mock Hollandaise Sauce

Ingredients

1- to-1 ¼-pounds asparagus

3 Tbsp reduced-fat mayonnaise

3 Tbsp reduced-sodium chicken or vegetable broth

2 Tbsp chopped fresh chives

¾ tsp grated lemon zest

1 Tbsp lemon juice

1 ½ tsp Dijon mustard

Pepper to taste

STEPS

1. To prepare, wash asparagus spears by holding them, tip ends down, under cold running water. Pat dry. Snap the tough end of spears off at the place where they break easily.
2. Place in steamer basket over boiling water. If trimmed asparagus spears are too long to fit in your steamer, cut them into 1 ½- to 2-inch lengths. Cover and steam until crisp-tender, 3 to 6 minutes.
3. Meanwhile, place reduced-fat mayonnaise in small saucepan. Gradually whisk in reduced-sodium chicken or vegetable broth. Set saucepan over medium-low heat; cook, whisking constantly, until heated through but not bubbling, about 2 minutes. Remove from heat. Stir in chives, lemon zest, lemon juice, Dijon mustard, and pepper. Spoon over hot asparagus.

Yield: 3 servings (3-4 oz asparagus, about 9 spears, and 2 tbsp sauce)
Per serving: 45 calories, 5g total fat, 0.5G saturated fat, 5g protein, 5g carbs, 3g fiber, 0mg cholesterol, 320mg sodium

100% Whole-Wheat Sandwich Bread

Ingredients

1 ½ cups warm water (100 to 110°F), divided, plus more
  for brushing over loaf and creating steam in oven
¾ tsp active dry yeast
3 ¼ to 3 ½ cups whole-wheat flour, divided
2 Tbsp molasses or honey
1 ½ tsp salt
Cooking spray
2 tsp cornmeal for coating loaf pan
1 Tbsp rolled oats for sprinkling over loaf

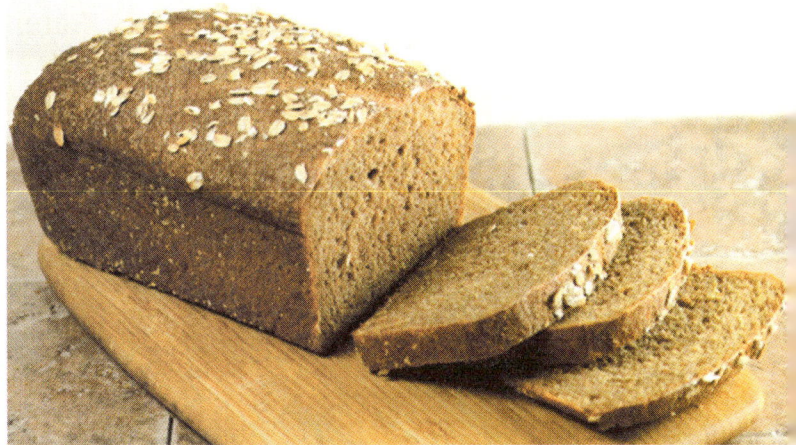

Steps

1. The day before baking, make "sponge": Place 1 cup water in large mixing bowl (use the bowl of your stand-up mixer if you have one). Sprinkle in yeast and let stand 5 minutes. Gradually add 1 ½ cups flour, whisking until well blended. Cover with plastic wrap and let stand at room temperature overnight, or until puffed and bubbly.
2. Stir together 1 ¼ cups flour and remaining ½ cup water in medium bowl until blended. Cover with plastic wrap and let the mixture stand overnight as well.
3. The following day, break flour-water mixture (from Step 2) into golf ball-size pieces and add to sponge mixture (from Step 1); mix with dough hook of stand-up mixer or manually with a wooden spoon. Add molasses and salt. Gradually beat in just enough additional flour until dough starts to pull away from sides of bowl. Knead with the dough hook or by hand on a lightly floured surface about 5 minutes, adding just enough additional flour to prevent sticking, or until smooth and springy.
4. Coat a large bowl with cooking spray. Place dough in bowl; turn to coat top. Cover with plastic wrap and let rise at room temperature 2 to 2 ½ hours, or until doubled. (Press two fingers into dough. If indentation remains, the dough has risen enough.)
5. Coat 8-by-4-inch loaf pan with cooking spray. Sprinkle with cornmeal. Turn dough out on to a lightly floured surface. Press dough into a rectangle. Fold short ends toward the center, then bring long sides together and pinch seam closed. Roll the log back and forth to make a smooth log shape. Place loaf, seam-side down, in prepared loaf pan. Spray a piece of plastic wrap with cooking spray and place, sprayed-side down, over loaf. Let rise at room temperature about 1 hour, or until almost doubled.
6. Meanwhile, about 20 minutes before baking, place metal baking pan on bottom shelf of oven and preheat oven to 375°F.
7. When you are ready to bake, brush top of loaf with a little water and sprinkle with rolled oats. Using a serrated knife, make a slash, about ¼-inch deep, down center of loaf (alternatively, make 3 diagonal slashes). Pour 1 cup water into baking pan in oven (steam in the oven helps the bread to rise). Place loaf pan on center shelf of oven and bake 20 minutes. Remove pan of water. Continue baking until loaf is golden brown and sounds hollow when tapped on the bottom, 15 to 25 minutes longer. Immediately remove loaf from pan and let cool completely on a wire rack before slicing.

Yield: 1 loaf
Per slice: 110 calories, 0.5G total fat, 0g saturated fat, 4g protein, 23g carbs, 3g fiber, 0mg cholesterol, 250mg sodium

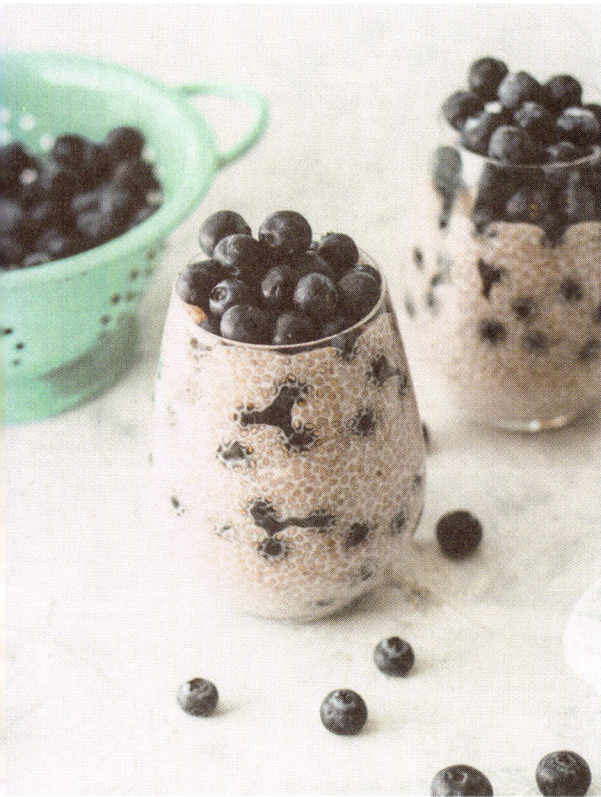

Blueberry-Chia Pudding

Ingredients

- ¼ cup chia seeds
- ½ cup unsweetened coconut milk
- ½ cup fresh blueberries
- 1 Tbsp honey
- ½ tsp vanilla extract

Steps

1. Combine chia seeds, honey, vanilla extract, and coconut milk. Stir to combine.
2. In a small bowl, lightly crush half of the blueberries and stir into the chia pudding. Gently stir in the remaining, whole blueberries.
3. Sit in the fridge, covered with plastic wrap for at least 30 minutes before serving.

Yield: 2 servings
Per serving: 170 calories, 8g total fat, 1.5G saturated fat, 4g protein, 23g carbs, 8g fiber, 0mg cholesterol, 3mg sodium
Source: Us Highbush Blueberry Council, Blueberrycouncil.org

Acetylcholine: A neurotransmitter in the parts of the brain involved in thinking, learning, and memory. Neurotransmitters are chemicals that allow cells in the brain to communicate with one another.

Alpha-linolenic acid (ALA): An essential fatty acid that, along with EPA and DHA, belongs to a group of fats called omega-3 fatty acids. EPA and DHA are found primarily in fish, while ALA is found in plant seeds and oils, such as flaxseed, canola, soy, walnuts, and walnut oils, and in wild plants like purslane. The body can convert ALA to EPA and DHA, which are more easily used by the body.

Alzheimer's disease: A form of dementia that progressively damages brain cells, leading to memory loss, personality changes, and other mental impairment. It is the most common form of dementia. (See: Dementia.)

Amino acids: The building blocks of proteins comprising 20 individual chemical units that are linked together in varying combinations.

Amyloid plaque: Protein pieces called beta-amyloid that clump together in the brains of people with Alzheimer's disease, which impair the ability of brain cells to function properly.

Amyloid precursor protein (APP): The beta-amyloid that clumps together to form amyloid plaques is a small piece of this larger protein.

Anthocyanins: A type of flavonoid in plants that acts as a pigment, giving many common fruits and vegetables their color.

Antioxidants: Substances that experts believe may protect cells from damage caused by unstable molecules known as free radicals, which are produced by the body as a normal byproduct of metabolism. Antioxidants include flavonoids, beta-carotene, lycopene, selenium, and vitamins A, C and E.

Atherosclerosis: Narrowing of the arteries due to an accumulation of fatty deposits and plaque.

Axon: An extension that carries impulses from one nerve cell to another.

Beta-amyloid: A chemically "sticky" protein that clumps together to form the plaques in the brain associated with Alzheimer's disease (See Amyloid plaque.)

Blood-brain barrier: A thin layer of cells that prevents potentially harmful substances from reaching the brain but allows essential nutrients to enter.

BMI: Body Mass Index, a calculation that combines weight and height: Weight in Pounds / (Height in inches x Height in inches) x 703. A BMI of over 25 is considered overweight, and over 30 is considered obese.

Carbohydrates: Compounds of carbon, hydrogen, and oxygen that form sugars, starches, and celluloses, mostly in plants, which provide energy for the body.

Cerebellum: The part of the brain related to movement, balance, and emotion.

Cerebral cortex: The gray, wrinkled layer that coats the surface of the brain's cerebrum and cerebellum, in which much of the brain's information processing occurs. The cerebral cortex is the outermost layer, and it is responsible for higher brain functions, such as intelligence, personality, planning, and organizing.

Cerebrum: The largest part of the brain, responsible for conscious mental processes, such as thinking, learning, and memory. The cerebrum is divided into left and right hemispheres ("left brain," "right brain").

Cholesterol: A waxy, fat-like substance found in foods of animal origin and synthesized by the body. Cholesterol is used for many of the body's processes, including hormone production. In large amounts in the blood, cholesterol can clog arteries.

Clinical trials: Research studies that test medical treatments in humans. The optimal clinical trials are randomized, placebo-controlled studies, meaning the participants are randomly assigned to treatment groups, and one group receives a placebo (inactive pill or device) and the other receives the study drug or device. In double-blind trials, neither the researchers nor the patients know which therapy any patient has received until the study is over. This removes any chance of bias in the results.

Cognition: Conscious intellectual activity, such as thinking and memory, orientation, language, judgment, and problem solving.

Cognitive decline: A loss of cognitive function, such as that associated with dementia.

Complex carbohydrates: Carbohydrates with three or more sugars, as opposed to simple carbohydrates composed of one or two sugars.

Creatine: An amino acid-like compound obtained naturally in the diet via high-protein foods, such as meat, fish, and eggs; the body also synthesizes creatine from amino acids.

CT scan (computed tomography): Computer-assisted scans that can assemble a static cross-section of the brain or other internal body area using X-rays. When assembled, the images provide a three-dimensional view of the area. People suspected of having dementia may have a CT scan of the brain to look for possible alternative causes of symptoms, such as a tumor or stroke.

Curcumin: The main component in the spice turmeric, undergoing study for its health benefits.

DASH diet: The Dietary Approaches to Stop Hypertension eating plan, high in fruits, vegetables, and grains, and low in meat, saturated fat, sweets, and salt. Study results suggest that you can lower high blood pressure with this eating plan.

Dementia: Umbrella term for a wide range of symptoms associated with a progressive decline in cognition that affect a person's ability to conduct everyday activities. There are several forms of dementia, the most common of which is Alzheimer's disease.

Docosahexaenoic acid (DHA): A type of fatty acid (omega-3 fatty acid) found in fish and algae that is essential for heart and brain health. (See: Eicosapentaenoic acid, and Omega-3 fatty acids.)

Eicosapentaenoic acid (EPA): A type of fatty acid (omega-3 fatty acid) found in fish that is essential for heart and brain health. (See: DHA, and Omega-3 fatty acids.)

Fats: Compounds containing fatty acids, which may be monounsaturated, polyunsaturated, or saturated.

Flavonoids: A group of more than 5,000 antioxidant compounds naturally present in vegetables, fruits, and beverages like tea, red wine, and fruit juices, and known for a dazzling array of pigments. Research suggests flavonoids may protect against damage to blood vessels, decreasing the risk of cardiovascular disease. In addition, they may have a role in cancer prevention and help boost the immune system.

fMRI scan: Functional magnetic resonance imaging, video scans that track the movement of oxygen-carrying hemoglobin to show blood flow in the brain.

Forebrain: The front-most of the three primary divisions of the brain, which contains the cerebrum and the structures that lie beneath it; responsible for the activities we call "thinking."

Frontal lobes: Twin brain structures, located behind the forehead, used for planning, weighing alternatives, and envisioning possible consequences; at the back of each frontal lobe, a motor area helps manage voluntary movement.

Frontotemporal dementia: One of several forms of dementia. The frontal and temporal anterior lobes of the brain shrink, which leads to either changes in behavior or problems with language.

Ginkgo biloba: A Chinese herbal remedy derived from the leaves of the ginkgo tree.

Glial cells: Material surrounding neurons, making up 90 percent of the brain's tissue.

Glucose: A sugar used by the body as a source of energy. For example, food is broken down in the digestive system into glucose.

Glycemic index (GI): A measure of how quickly the body converts a food to blood sugar (glucose) after eating a specific amount of a food when compared to the same amount of a control food, usually glucose or white bread. The number indicating the rise in blood sugar is called the "glycemic index." The faster the carbohydrate from a food enters the bloodstream, the greater the increase in insulin levels, and the higher its glycemic index.

Glycemic load: Measure that compares a food's glycemic index with typical serving size, calories, and carbohydrates.

Hemorrhagic stroke: A stroke caused by the leakage of blood out of a blood vessel into the brain.

High blood pressure: Blood pressure measures the force of blood against the artery walls. High blood pressure is force at an abnormally high level.

High-density lipoprotein (HDL) cholesterol: A type of lipoprotein particle that carries "bad" (LDL) cholesterol from your tissues to the liver for excretion. HDL-C is "good" cholesterol and reduces cholesterol buildup in the arteries. High levels of HDL are desirable, because they are linked with a reduced risk of cardiovascular disease that can lead to heart attack or stroke. (See: Cholesterol, Low-density lipoprotein [LDL] cholesterol.)

Hindbrain: The rearmost of the three primary divisions of the brain; it includes the upper spinal cord, brainstem, and cerebellum, and controls the body's vital functions, such as the heart rate and breathing.

Hippocampus: A structure in the brain that is involved in short- and long-term memory. In people with Alzheimer's disease the hippocampus shrinks considerably.

Homocysteine: An amino acid in the blood that is a marker of cardiovascular disease risk.

Huperzine A: A moss extract used as a Chinese herbal remedy.

Hypertension: High blood pressure. Known as "the silent killer," hypertension is a very important risk factor for stroke and heart attack as well as other disorders.

Hypothalamus: Area of the inner brain that controls waking, adrenaline, and the molecules that incite emotions.

Inflammation: The response of body tissues to injury or irritation. Inflammation (swelling) occurs when trauma, bacteria, heat, or other causes injure tissues of the body. This is a response of the immune system that helps rid the body of foreign substances and aids in healing. Sometimes inflammation persists beyond the time when it is useful and it can become harmful.

Ischemic stroke: A stroke caused when a blocked blood vessel to the brain starves the brain tissue of oxygen.

Lewy body: Abnormal aggregates of protein that develop inside nerve cells in Parkinson's disease (PD), dementia with Lewy bodies, and some other neurological disorders.

Lewy body dementia: One of several forms of dementia. Lewy bodies are microscopic proteins that can accumulate in the brain and cause mental decline. People with this type of dementia also have other symptoms, such as drowsiness, lethargy, visual hallucinations, physical rigidity, and loss of spontaneous movement.

Lipid: A word used to encompass many different kinds of fat-soluble molecules, including cholesterol, triglycerides, and free fatty acids.

Lipoprotein: A specialized, microscopic, spherical particle in the blood composed of protein and lipids. Its role is to move lipids from one part of the body to another.

Low-density lipoprotein (LDL) cholesterol: A type of lipoprotein particle that carries cholesterol to the tissues, where it can build up in the liver and lead to heart disease. LDL-C is "bad" cholesterol. (See: Cholesterol, High-density lipoprotein [HDL] cholesterol.)

Lycopene: The natural red pigment that gives tomatoes, red bell peppers, watermelon, and other fruits and vegetables their color. Research suggests it is a powerful antioxidant that may aid in preventing heart disease and several types of cancer. Cooked tomato products contain the form of lycopene that is easiest for the body to absorb and utilize.

Magnetic resonance imaging (MRI): An imaging technique that uses magnetic fields instead of x-rays to create images of internal structures in the body, including the brain, heart, and other organs.

Mediterranean diet: A dietary pattern similar to that traditionally found in areas around the Mediterranean Sea in countries such as Greece, southern Italy, and Spain. It emphasizes olive oil as the primary source of dietary fat, an abundance of plant foods, including fruits, vegetables, whole grains, beans, nuts, and seeds, and moderate amounts of fish, poultry, dairy foods, and wine. The Mediterranean diet is low in red meat and saturated fats and contains no added sugars or processed foods.

Midbrain: The middle of the three primary divisions of the brain; it includes the uppermost part of the brainstem. The midbrain controls some of your reflexes and is involved in coordinating eye movements and other voluntary motions.

Mild cognitive impairment (MCI): Problems with memory, thinking, and other cognitive functions that are more pronounced than normal age-related changes but don't interfere with daily functioning; having MCI raises the risk for developing dementia.

Mini-Mental State Examination (MMSE): A brief, 30-item questionnaire used to screen for cognitive impairment; also known as the Folstein test.

Modified Mini-Mental State Examination (3MS): A widely used screening test for dementia that is an expanded form of the Mini-Mental State Examination (MMSE).

Monounsaturated fat: A type of healthy fat in which only one carbon atom is not bound to hydrogen (this is also called a "double bond"); monounsaturated fats, found in olive, walnut, canola, and other vegetable oils, are generally liquid at room temperature.

Myelin: A fatty substance that surrounds and insulates the nerves.

Neurofibrillary tangles: Dense proteins within nerve cells in the brain that injure the cells. The tangles are twisted threads, the major component of which is a protein called tau. Along with amyloid plaques, these are a hallmark of Alzheimer's disease.

Neurons: Nerve cells that transmit electrical and chemical messages via the nervous system throughout the brain, spinal cord, and body.

Neurotransmitter: A chemical substance produced by the body that acts as a messenger in the brain and nervous system by transmitting nerve impulses from one cell to another cell, muscle, tissue, or organ; examples include dopamine, epinephrine, and serotonin. Neurotransmitters play an essential role in the normal functioning of the brain.

Omega-3 fatty acids: Unsaturated fats found in fish, walnuts, flaxseeds, and some other plant foods that are associated with disease prevention. Diets rich in omega-3s have been linked with a reduced risk of cardiovascular disease and depression, as well as improved brain function.

Omega-6 fatty acids: A type of unsaturated fat found in many nuts, seeds, and vegetable oils, and in some poultry, seafood, and vegetables. One omega-6 fatty acid, linoleic acid, is essential because the body requires it but cannot make it, and must derive it through diet.

PET scan (positron emission tomography): A test that tracks signals given off by a radioactive substance that has been injected into a vein, producing three-dimensional images of internal organs and tissues.

Phosphatidylserine (PS): A fat-like substance found in cell membranes, especially in the human brain, that supports healthy cognitive function. A form of PS has been extracted from soybeans and sold as a supplement that claims to improve memory, although research has not confirmed its effectiveness.

Phytochemicals (also called phytonutrients): Compounds in plants that provide flavor, aroma, and color, and protect the plant from microbes and environmental damage. When consumed by humans, phytochemicals are believed to promote health and prevent disease. Many phytochemicals are antioxidants.

Placebo: An inactive substance used in randomized, controlled scientific studies, usually when testing medications. Study participants who receive placebos are the "control group," and their data are compared with data from participants who are taking the medication being studied. However, study participants are "blind," meaning they are not told if they are taking a placebo or a medication.

Plaque: Fatty deposits that form on the inside surface of arteries that are characteristic of atherosclerosis; plaque may contain lipids (including cholesterol), calcium, white blood cells, and blood clots (See Amyloid plaque).

Plasticity: The ability of the brain to reorganize itself by developing new neural connections throughout a person's life; also called neuroplasticity.

Polyphenols: A group of naturally occurring plant compounds, including flavonoids and isoflavones, with antioxidant properties that may benefit health.

Polyunsaturated fat: A type of healthy fat in which more than one carbon atom is not bound to hydrogen; polyunsaturated fats found in soybean, corn, sunflower, and other vegetable oils are generally liquid at room temperature.

Protein kinase C (PKC): An enzyme in the brain that affects the prefrontal cortex.

Protein: An essential component of all living cells. Dietary protein supplies the body with essential amino acids needed for formation, growth, and repair of cells and tissues in muscles, bones, blood, and skin, as well as the production of enzymes and hormones.

Resveratrol: This naturally occurring phytonutrient is mainly found in the skins of red grapes (and therefore in red wine) and in lesser amounts in the skins of peanuts. Researchers are exploring its potential anti-aging, antioxidant, and cancer-fighting properties.

Saturated fat: A type of fat in which all carbon atoms are bound to hydrogen, and that can increase unhealthy cholesterol levels and raise the risk of heart disease. Saturated fatty acids are found primarily in animal foods, especially meats and full-fat dairy products. They are generally solid at room temperature, as in butter or lard, and are the chief culprit in unhealthy blood cholesterol levels. Saturated fat is also found in a few vegetable products such as coconut, palm, and palm kernel oils.

Simple carbohydrates: Carbohydrates containing one (single) or two (double) sugars, as opposed to complex carbohydrates, which have three or more sugars. Found in refined white flour, white rice, candy, non-diet carbonated beverages, syrups, and table sugar.

Stroke: An acute vascular event that occurs in the brain, most often caused by a blood clot that lodges in an artery and blocks the flow of blood to the brain (ischemic stroke), producing symptoms ranging from limb paralysis and loss of speech to unconsciousness and death. Less commonly, a stroke may be caused by bleeding into the brain (hemorrhagic stroke).

Synapse: Junction points that connect neurons and other nerve cells.

Systolic pressure: The pressure of the blood in the arteries when the heart contracts. It is the higher of two blood pressure measurements. For example, in a blood pressure reading of 120/80 mm Hg, 120 is the systolic pressure.

Tangle: In Alzheimer's disease, a collapsed group of tau proteins that disrupts the flow of nutrients to part of the brain.

Tau: A type of protein that, in a healthy brain, carries essential nutrients; in Alzheimer's disease, tangles of collapsed tau proteins disrupt this flow.

Temporal lobes: Twin areas, under the parietal and frontal lobes of the brain, that process input from the ears, as well as integrating sensory input and memories.

Thalamus: The part of the brain that relays impulses, especially sensory impulses from the nerves, and enables people to feel pain.

Thrombotic stroke: A stroke resulting when a blood clot (thrombus) stops the flow of blood in an artery leading to or in the brain.

Trans fat: A type of fat that is manufactured by adding hydrogen to liquid oil to solidify it, resulting in the formation of partially hydrogenated oil. Trans fat increases unhealthy LDL cholesterol levels and lowers healthy HDL cholesterol levels.

Triglycerides: A form of fat found in food, fat tissue, and the bloodstream; calories you consume that are not used immediately by the body's tissues are converted to triglycerides and transported to fat cells to be stored. Elevated triglycerides in the bloodstream are a risk factor for heart disease.

Unsaturated fat: A type of fatty acid that lowers cholesterol levels and reduces the risk for coronary artery disease especially when it is consumed in place of saturated and trans fats. Monounsaturated and polyunsaturated fatty acids fall into this category.

Vascular dementia: Dementia caused by blood vessel damage in the brain; it is the second-most common form of dementia after Alzheimer's disease.

Vegan: A diet that eliminates all animal products, including dairy, eggs, and honey.

Vegetarian: A diet that eliminates meat, but still may include dairy and eggs. Vegetarians who consume fish are called pescatarians.

Vinpocetine: A synthetic compound made to resemble a substance found naturally in the periwinkle plant, used for stroke and Alzheimer's prevention, and for other disorders, such as chronic fatigue syndrome and symptoms of menopause.

Whole grains: Grains that contain all the essential parts and naturally occurring nutrients of the entire grain seed—the bran, germ, and endosperm.

Alzheimer's Association
www.alz.org
800-272-3900
225 N. Michigan Avenue, Floor 17
Chicago, IL 60601-7633

Alzheimer's Drug Discovery Foundation
www.alzdiscovery.org
212-901-8000
57 West 57th Street, Suite 904
New York, NY 10019

Alzheimer's Foundation of America
www.alzfdn.org
866-AFA-8484
322 8th Avenue, 7th Floor
New York, NY 10001

**Association for Frontotemporal
Degeneration (AFTD)**
866-507-7222
www.theaftd.org
Radnor Station Building #2, Suite 320
290 King of Prussia Road
Radnor, PA 19087

**Friedman School of Nutrition Science and
Policy—Tufts University**
nutrition.tufts.edu
617-636-3777
150 Harrison Avenue
Boston, MA 02111

**Jean Mayer USDA Human Nutrition
Research Center of Aging**
hnrca.tufts.edu
617-556-3000
711 Washington Street
Boston, MA 02111

Lewy Body Dementia Association
www.lbda.org
800-539-9767
912 Killian Hill Road, S.W.
Lilburn, GA 30047

**National Center for Complementary
and Integrative Health**
nccih.nih.gov
888-644-6226

National Family Caregivers Association
www.thefamilycaregiver.org
800-896-3650
10400 Connecticut Avenue, Suite 500
Kensington, MD 20895-3944

**National Institute on Aging
Alzheimer's Disease Education
and Referral Center**
www.nia.nih.gov/alzheimers
800-438-4380
Building 31, Room 5C27
31 Center Drive, MSC 2292
Bethesda, MD 20892

Medline Plus
www.nlm.nih.gov/medlineplus

**National Institute of Neurological
Disorders and Stroke
NIH Neurological Institute**
800-352-9424
www.ninds.nih.gov
P.O. Box 5801
Bethesda, MD 20824

**National Institute of Mental Health (NIMH)
National Institutes of Health, DHHS**
www.nimh.nih.gov
866-415-8051
6001 Executive Boulevard, Room 8184, MSC 9663
Bethesda, MD 20892-9663

Tufts University Health & Nutrition Letter
www.nutritionletter.tufts.edu

USDA Choose My Plate
www.choosemyplate.gov
888-779-7264

Whole Grains Council
www.wholegrainscouncil.org
617-421-5500
266 Beacon Street
Boston, MA 02116